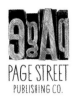

First published in 2023 by
Page Street Publishing Co.
27 Congress Street, Suite 1511
Salem, MA 01970
www.pagestreetpublishing.com

Distributed by Macmillan, sales in Canada by The Canadian Manda Group.

27 26 25 24 23   1 2 3 4 5

ISBN-13: 978-1-64567-965-3
ISBN-10: 1-64567-965-9

Library of Congress Control Number: 2022921013

Cover and book design by Laura Benton for Page Street Publishing Co.
Photography by Bjorn Bolinder and Find The Light Photography
Inspiration Images by Yogi Beans, Adobe Stock, Unsplash

Printed and bound in China

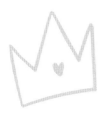

TO ViViENNE AND JULiETTE

**MAY YOU ALWAYS SEE THE WORLD THROUGH EYES
OF WONDER AND WiTH AN OPEN HEART**

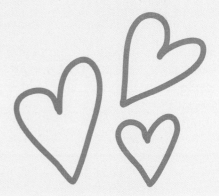

CONTENTS

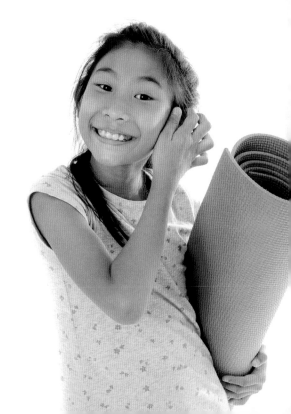

Namaste, Kids!

Welcome to the wonderful world of yoga! Did you know that *yoga* is an ancient practice that originated in India a . . .

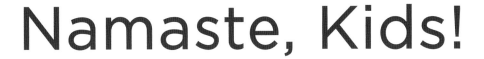

Really, Really, REALLY, LONG TiME AGO

People have been practicing yoga for thousands of years because it can help us FEEL GOOD! You can think of yoga as exercise for your body, mind and heart.

We are excited for you to begin your yoga journey, and we hope this book gives you an opportunity to explore—and notice—how different yoga poses make you feel. By moving through the poses in this book, you will discover that yoga is physically engaging, makes your body feel good and can be loads of fun!

Lauren & Brian

YOU CAN USE THIS BOOK IN A FEW DIFFERENT WAYS:

PRACTICE ONE POSE A DAY. This can be a joyful way to begin each day or to do at the end of the day before you go to bed—or anytime you like. You will have enough poses for 3 months!

CHOOSE ONE THEME EACH WEEK. Notice how different the poses feel from the beginning of the week to the end.

PRACTICE WITH A FRIEND, SIBLING OR GROWN-UP. One person reads the "Who Am I?" clue aloud and the other person guesses the answer to the clue. Then, practice the pose together!

PARTNER POSES. Practice the partner poses (pages 130 to 135) with a friend, sibling or grown-up!

If you come across words in purple, these words are *Sanskrit*, the ancient language of South Asia, where yoga evolved from. Use the Glossary on page 138 to look up the meaning of these words as you discover them!

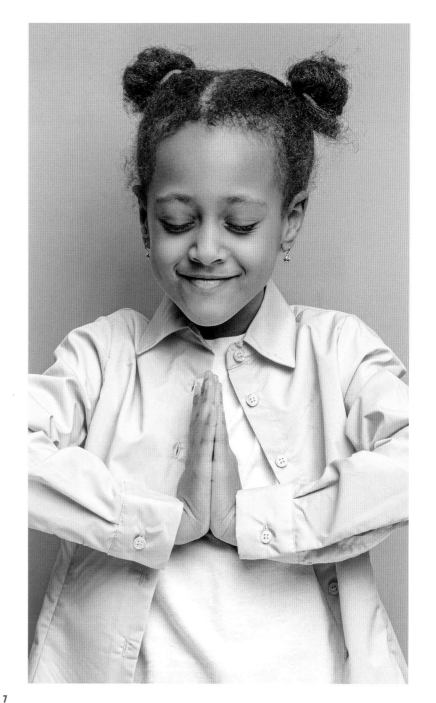

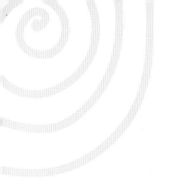
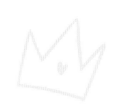

Begin with the Breath

While this book focuses mainly on yoga poses (***asanas***), the breath (***pranayama***) is an important part of any yoga practice. I imagine at some point in your life you may have been told to "take a deep breath." When you change the way you breathe, you can change the way you feel.

Deep, slow and long breaths can help us feel more calm and supported. As you move through the poses in this book, remember to pay attention to the connection between your breath and your body. Do you notice your breathing patterns change as you practice different poses? For example, do you hold your breath when practicing a pose that feels more challenging? Try to use your breath to help soften and ease into each pose.

Think of your breath as a friend who is always with you and helps you feel more comfortable and relaxed in challenging situations.

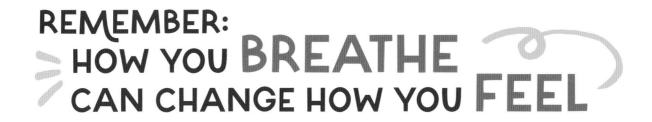

REMEMBER:
HOW YOU BREATHE
CAN CHANGE HOW YOU FEEL

Why 108?

You may be wondering why we chose 108 yoga poses in this book. 108 is a special number in many religions and traditions (including yoga), as well as in geometry, arithmetic, astrology and numerology. The number 108 has been called "nature's secret code" or "nature's universal rule."

Mathematicians of the **Vedic** culture believe the number 108 has a way of representing the wholeness of existence. Below are a few examples of how the number 108 shows up in our world:

- The distance from the Earth to the Sun is about 108 times the diameter of the Sun.

- The distance between the Earth and the Moon is also about 108 times the diameter of the Moon.

- There are 108 beads on an Indian **mala** necklace.

- There are 108 pressure points on the body in **Ayurveda** and traditional Chinese medicine.

- In astrology, there are 12 constellations and 9 arc segments (12 x 9 = 108).

- There are 108 stitches on a baseball!

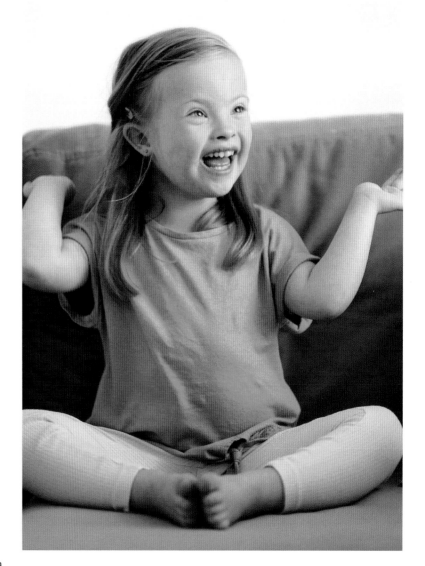

Namaste, Adults!

Yogi Beans is all about the vibration of yoga! This book is a visual guide to 108 poses across different themes. You can use this book with your children, students or patients as a way to incorporate yoga into their daily lives.

For adults that teach children's yoga, you can use this book as a guide to cueing and teaching yoga poses as well as learning how to group poses into different themes to create novel thematic experiences for children.

Most importantly, when practicing yoga with children, keep the energy light and playful!

REMEMBER: YOGA iS A PRACTICE, NOT A PERFECT!

HOW TO USE THiS BOOK

Each pose contains the following information on how to best use and present yoga poses to children:

LET'S MOVE: Child-friendly cues to help children move efficiently through the poses. Remember to practice each movement on both sides of the body.

ANATOMiCAL FOCUS: The specific part of anatomy targeted in each pose

POSE TYPE: Category of the pose (e.g., seated, standing)

SANSKRiT NAME: The traditional Sanskrit name of the yoga pose. For some poses, we use the word "variation" in the Sanskrit name to denote a nontraditional pose that is partially based on a classic yoga pose. Any creative movement-based pose does not have a Sanskrit name.

AGE: Recommended minimum age to introduce the pose (e.g., 2+). Age recommendations are based on our experience teaching yoga to children and are not strict requirements.

VALUE: The correlative value for a pose expressed in an "I AM" affirmation

WHAT/WHO AM I? POSE DESCRIPTiONS: Near the name of each pose is a description of an animal or object. We encourage you to read these descriptions out loud so children have an opportunity to guess the pose prior to practicing it (without peeking at the book)!

POSE TRANSiTiONS: Some poses lead into other poses. In such instances, we indicate the page that shows the first pose such as, "Begin in Mountain pose (page 19)."

BEAN TiPS: You'll see these tips and tricks for different poses to help you practice.

We trust this book provides you with a valuable resource that enables you to share the practice of yoga with children in your home, yoga studio, classroom or clinic.

BONUS CONTENT

Scan the QR code below to unlock bonus digital content to accompany this book! There you will find a child-friendly printable Sun Salutation sequence, as well as discounts to Yogi Beans video content.

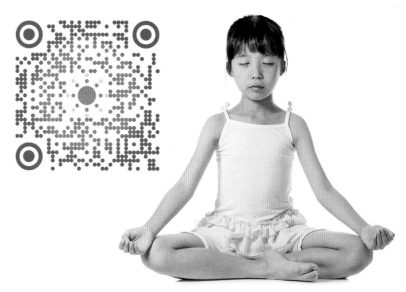

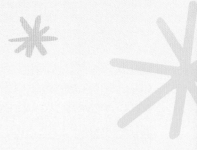

STARTING
POSES
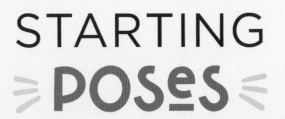

Are you ready to start your yoga adventure?! Before you dive in, it is helpful to learn some of the **most commonly practiced poses**. You may actually know some of these poses already! Notice how you feel as you move into each pose, and try not to jump to any **conclusions** or **judgements**.

REMEMBER THE YOGI BEANS AFFIRMATION:
It is a yoga practice—not a yoga perfect!

Let's play and have some yoga fun together!

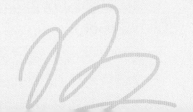

Downward Dog

Adho Mukha Svanasana

I wag my tail **back** and **forth** when I am happy.

LET'S MOVE!

With your hands firmly planted on the ground, **lift** your tailbone up high and **give your tail a wiggle**. Peddle your feet as if you are a dog going for a walk in your favorite park.

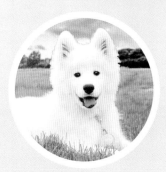

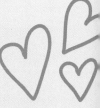

AGE: 2+

POSE TYPE: Inversion

ANATOMICAL FOCUS: Legs, Arms

VALUE: I AM friendly

13

Cat

Marjaryasana

WHO AM I?

I **purr** when I am feeling happy and relaxed. I like to **rub** my head and neck on **people I love.**

LET'S MOVE!

On your hands and knees, look down at your belly button and **round** your back like a scared cat on Halloween. **Let out a cute meow!**

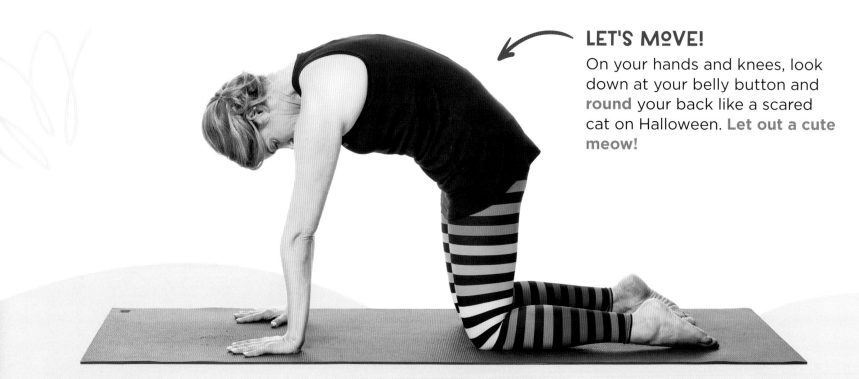

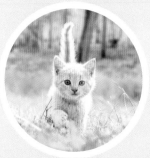

AGE: 2+

POSE TYPE: Core

ANATOMICAL FOCUS: Back

VALUE: I AM coordinated

Cow
Bitilasana

WHO AM I?

I am a **sacred animal** in India (yoga's birthplace). I also produce **milk.**

LET'S MOVE!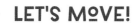

Begin on all fours and drop your belly (these are your udders). **Gaze up** to the sky and let out a **loud moo!**

BEAN TIP: In yoga, Cat pose and Cow pose are **best friends.** They are often practiced together!

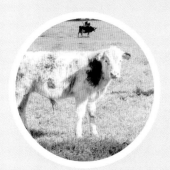

AGE: 2+

POSE TYPE: Backbend

ANATOMICAL FOCUS: Back

VALUE: I AM nourished

Cobra

Bhujangasana

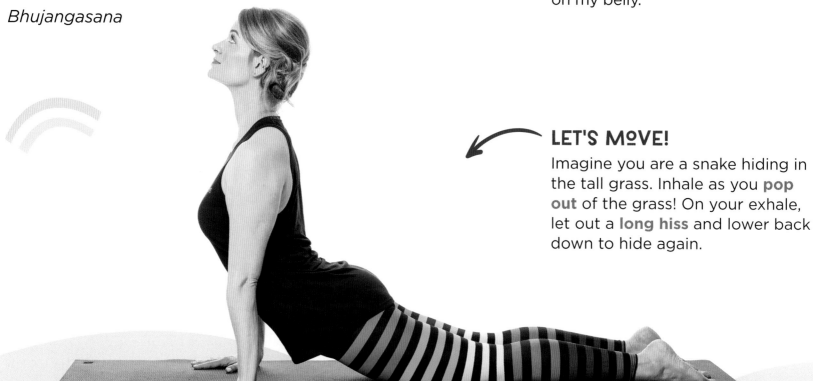

WHO AM I?

I have **no legs** and I **slither** around on my belly.

LET'S MOVE!

Imagine you are a snake hiding in the tall grass. Inhale as you **pop out** of the grass! On your exhale, let out a **long hiss** and lower back down to hide again.

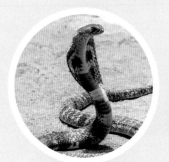

AGE: 2+

POSE TYPE: Backbend

ANATOMICAL FOCUS: Back

VALUE: I AM powerful

Mouse

(Also called Child's Pose)

Balasana

WHO AM I?

I love cheese! I say **"squeak!"**

BEAN TIP: Mouse pose is great to practice any time you are feeling overwhelmed and need a break.

LET'S MOVE!

Come onto your knees and sit back on your heels. Bend forward and bring your forehead to the floor. Can you be as **quiet as a mouse** and rest in this pose for **three slow breaths?**

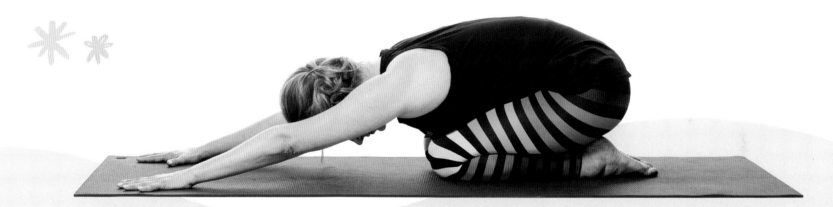

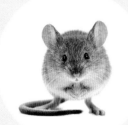

AGE: 2+

POSE TYPE: Forward Bend

ANATOMICAL FOCUS: Legs, Back

VALUE: I AM attentive

Upward Facing Dog

Urdvha Mukha Svanasana

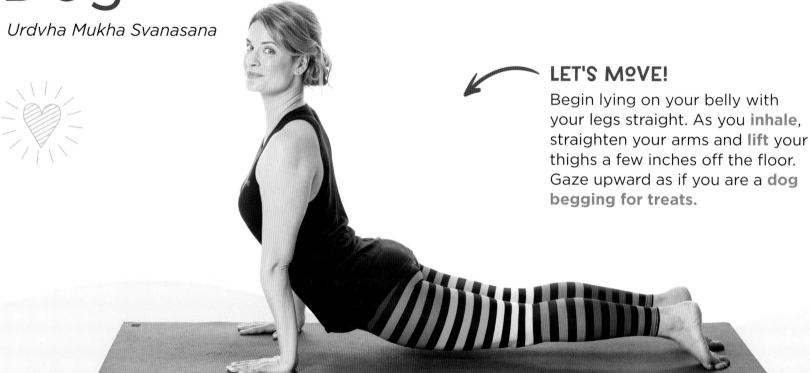

WHO AM I?

I am a downward facing dog turned **upside down!**

LET'S MOVE!

Begin lying on your belly with your legs straight. As you **inhale**, straighten your arms and **lift** your thighs a few inches off the floor. Gaze upward as if you are a **dog begging for treats.**

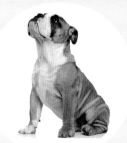

AGE: 8+

POSE TYPE: Backbend

ANATOMICAL FOCUS: Back, Chest

VALUE: I AM joyful

Mountain

Tadasana

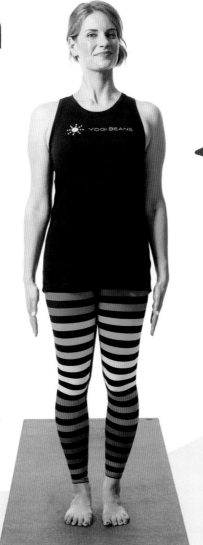

WHAT AM I?

I am **taller** than a hill and I have a **sharp** peak. People like **skiing** down me when it snows.

LET'S MOVE!

Stand straight with your hands at your side. Your mountain is **strong** and nothing can **knock you down!** Can you hold this position and remain silent and still while taking a deep breath?

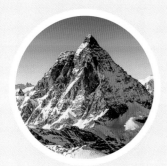

AGE: 2+

POSE TYPE: Standing

ANATOMICAL FOCUS: Legs, Back

VALUE: I AM stable

Triangle

Utthita Trikonasana

WHAT AM I?

I am the shape of a slice of **pizza** or a slice of **watermelon**. I have three sides.

BEAN TIP: Practice this pose with a friend or in front of a mirror. Count how many triangles you can spot in the pose!

LET'S MOVE!

From Proud Warrior pose (page 64), straighten your front leg. **Tip over like a teapot** and place your front hand on your leg, foot or floor (whichever is most comfortable).

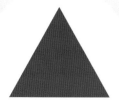

AGE: 3+

POSE TYPE: Standing

ANATOMICAL FOCUS: Legs

VALUE: I AM intentional

Right Angle

Utthita Parsvakonasana

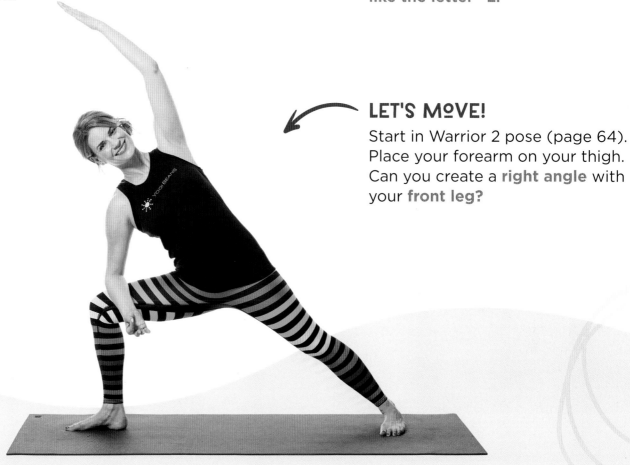

WHAT AM I?

I can be the corner of a room or the corner of a book. **I am shaped like the letter "L."**

LET'S MOVE!

Start in Warrior 2 pose (page 64). Place your forearm on your thigh. Can you create a **right angle** with your **front leg?**

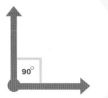

AGE: 5+

POSE TYPE: Standing

ANATOMICAL FOCUS: Legs

VALUE: I AM supported

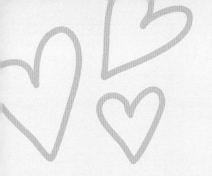

OLD McYOGI'S
FARM

You may have heard of **Old McDonald**, but are you familiar with his cousin **Old McYogi**? Old McYogi is also a farmer who has great compassion for all the animals that live on the farm. **Hop on your tractor** and learn which animals call Old McYogi's farm their home.

Pony

Eka Pada Adho Mukha Svanasana

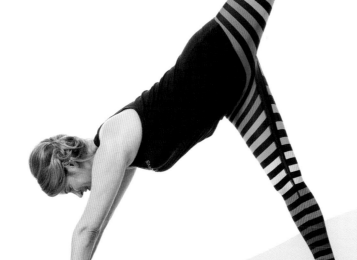

WHO AM I?

I can **walk, trot, canter** and **gallop!**

LET'S MOVE!

Begin in Downward Dog (page 13) and lift one leg high into the air. Imagine your leg is your pony tail and **let out a "neigh!"**

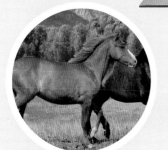

AGE: 2+

POSE TYPE: Inversion

ANATOMICAL FOCUS: Legs

VALUE: I AM free

Pig

WHO AM I?

On a hot day, I like to **roll in the mud** to stay cool.

LET'S MOVE!

While lying flat on your back, circle your arms and legs and pretend to be a pig **playing in the mud.** Do you feel this pose in your center when you **tuck** your chin and **lift** your head off the floor?

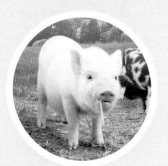

AGE: 2+

POSE TYPE: Core

ANATOMICAL FOCUS: Legs, Core

VALUE: I AM compassionate

Rabbit

Sasangasana Variation

WHO AM I?

I have long ears and a fluffy tail.
I hop around!

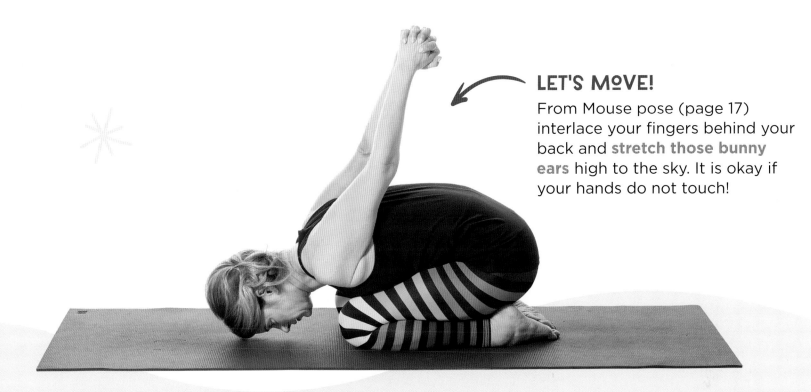

LET'S MOVE!

From Mouse pose (page 17) interlace your fingers behind your back and **stretch those bunny ears** high to the sky. It is okay if your hands do not touch!

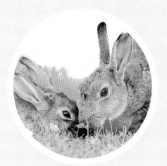

AGE: 5+

POSE TYPE: Forward Bend

ANATOMICAL FOCUS: Shoulders

VALUE: I AM empathetic

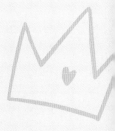

Frog

Malasana

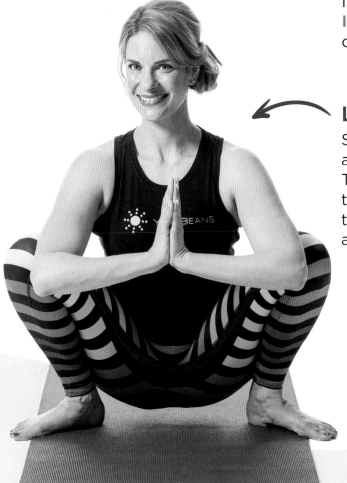

WHO AM I?

I am an amphibian that lives on **land** and in **water.** I start my life cycle as a **tadpole.**

LET'S MOVE!

Squat down low with your hands at heart center and take a breath. Then, **hop like a frog!** Can you take **ten** frog jumps? Try counting to ten in another language for added fun.

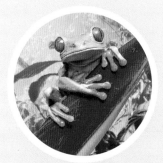

AGE: 2+

POSE TYPE: Standing

ANATOMICAL FOCUS: Legs

VALUE: I AM transformative

Bull

Gomukhasana

BEAN TIP: To switch sides, keep your feet firmly planted and pivot to the other side. We call this a "bull whirl!"

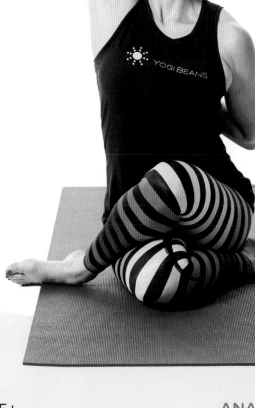

WHO AM I?

I am an adult male cow with **large feet,** a **muscular neck** and **thick bones.** I can get very **mad.**

LET'S MOVE!

Place one knee over the other. **Keep your spine long** and extend your hand overhead to place your palm on your back. Now, **reach** your opposite arm behind your back. See if you can hold your hands.

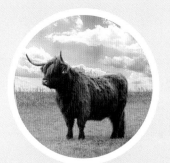

AGE: 5+

POSE TYPE: Seated

ANATOMICAL FOCUS: Hips, Shoulders

VALUE: I AM strong

Goat

Malasana Variation

WHO AM I?

I am very **intelligent** and **curious**. The sound I make when speaking is called a **bleat.**

LET'S MOVE!

Squat down low and try to keep your heels pressed together. **Stretch** your arms out long in front of you. **Imagine** your knees are your **goat ears!**

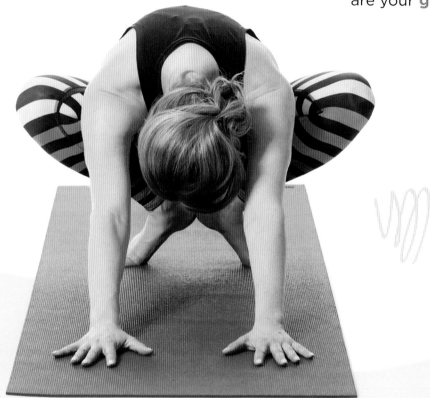

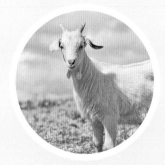

AGE: 3+

POSE TYPE: Standing

ANATOMICAL FOCUS: Hips, Back

VALUE: I AM creative

Lamb

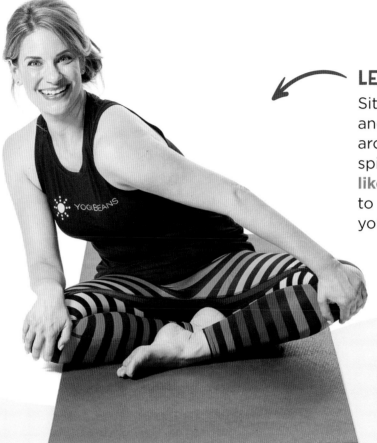

WHO AM I?

I travel in **flocks** and my coat is made of **fluffy wool.**

LET'S MOVE!

Sit cross-legged on your mat and circle the top of your body around as if you are wool on a spinning wheel. **Say "baaah" like a little lamb.** Remember to switch the direction of your circles!

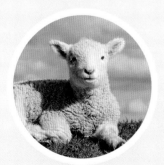

AGE: 2+

POSE TYPE: Seated

ANATOMICAL FOCUS: Hips, Back

VALUE: I AM gentle

Plow

Halasana

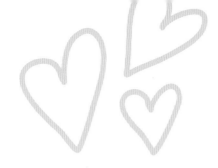

WHAT AM I?

I am a **tool** used by a farmer to loosen the soil before **planting crops.**

BEAN TIP: Remember, stay on your shoulders—**never roll onto your neck**—when you are in this pose.

LET'S MOVE!

Lie on your back with your arms by your side, palms facing down. Bring your legs **up and over and behind** your head.

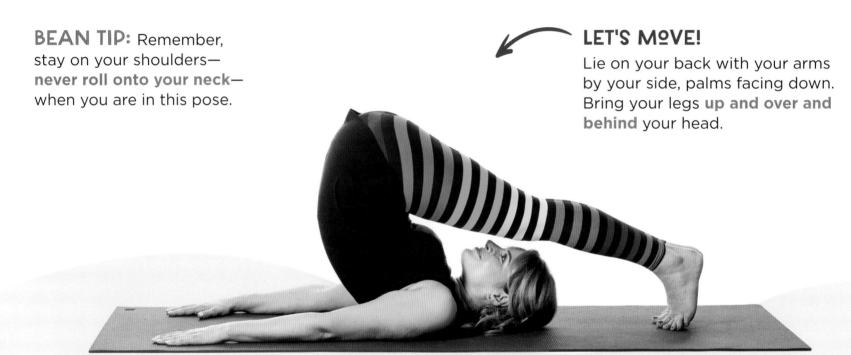

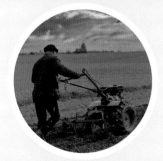

AGE: 3+

POSE TYPE: Inversion

ANATOMICAL FOCUS: Back, Legs

VALUE: I AM of service

Windmill

Parivrtta Prasarita Padottanasana

WHAT AM I?

I am a **large machine** powered by the **wind** to produce **electricity.**

BEAN TIP: Make sure your hand crosses over your belly button to touch the opposite foot.

LET'S MOVE!

Begin standing in a wide straddle. Cross your hand over your belly button to touch the opposite foot. Repeat on the other side. **Imagine it is windy outside** and have fun speeding up the pose!

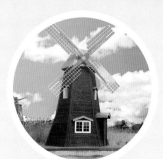

AGE: 3+

POSE TYPE: Twist

ANATOMICAL FOCUS: Legs, Back

VALUE: I AM sustainable

WILD SAFARI
RIDE

Rise and shine! Early morning is the best time to go on a wild safari ride! You'll observe some of your favorite animals in their natural habitats as you watch the sun **rise** and **light up** the sky. Don't forget to bring your binoculars!

Tiger

Vyaghrasana

WHO AM I?

I am the **largest cat** in the world. You will know who I am by seeing my **orange coat and dark stripes.**

LET'S MOVE!

This pose can be done kneeling or in Plank pose (page 90). As you **lift your leg** in the air, imagine you are a **crouching tiger** that is getting ready to **pounce!**

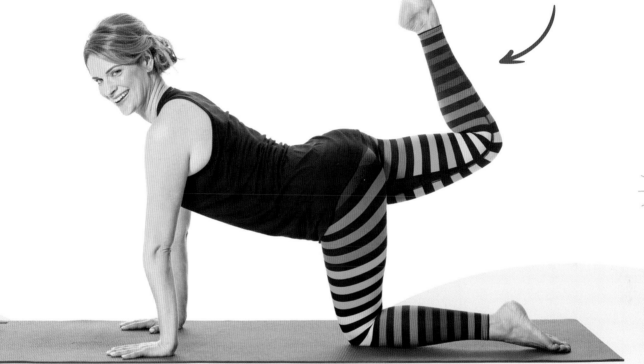

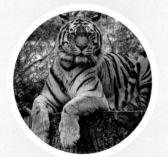

AGE: 5+

POSE TYPE: Core

ANATOMICAL FOCUS: Legs, Core

VALUE: I AM confident

Lion's Breath

Simhasana

WHO AM I?
I am the **King of the Jungle!**

BEAN TIP: Lion's breath is a helpful tool when you are feeling **mad or frustrated.** A big lion's breath can help make your anger feel a little bit smaller.

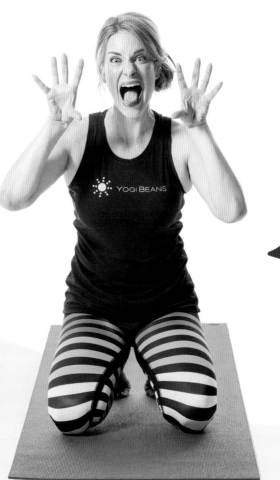

LET'S MOVE!

Scratch your lion paws, stick out your lion chest and inhale deeply. On your exhale, let out a **big roar** and **stick out your tongue!**

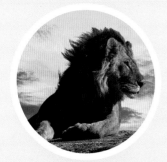

AGE: 2+

POSE TYPE: Seated, Breathing

ANATOMICAL FOCUS: Breath

VALUE: I AM courageous

Monkey

Ardha Hanumanasana

WHO AM I?

I am a primate with opposable thumbs. I can be **mischievous** and **playful.** I love to **swing in the trees.**

BEAN TIP: If you are feeling very flexible, try coming into a full split from this pose. Notice if one side feels different than the other.

LET'S MOVE!

Begin in a lunge with one knee on the ground. Place your hands on the floor and slowly straighten your leg. **Monkey sounds are encouraged!**

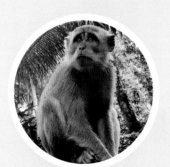

AGE: 5+

POSE TYPE: Seated

ANATOMICAL FOCUS: Legs

VALUE: I AM intelligent

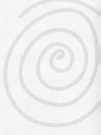

Giraffe

Urdhva Hastasana

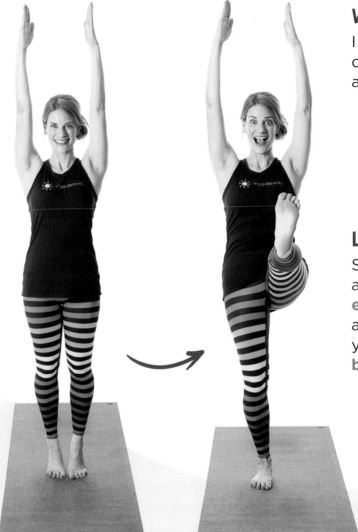

WHO AM I?

I am the **tallest** land mammal on **Earth.** Did you know that I also have a **bluish tongue?**

LET'S MOVE!

Stretch your arms up high and **imagine you are a giraffe eating leaves** from the top of a tall tree. Practice kicking your long legs and take some **big** giraffe steps.

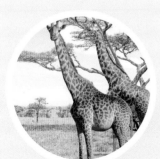

AGE: 2+

POSE TYPE: Standing

ANATOMICAL FOCUS: Legs

VALUE: I AM kind

Zebra

Prasarita Padottanasana Variation

WHO AM I?

I have a unique pattern of **black** and **white stripes.**

LET'S MOVE!

From Mountain pose (page 19), **jump your legs out** into a straddle. Stretch both arms out in front of you to form a pair of **"stripes."**

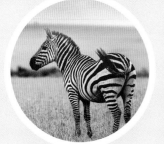

AGE: 2+

POSE TYPE: Forward Bend

ANATOMICAL FOCUS: Legs, Back

VALUE: I AM unique

Elephant

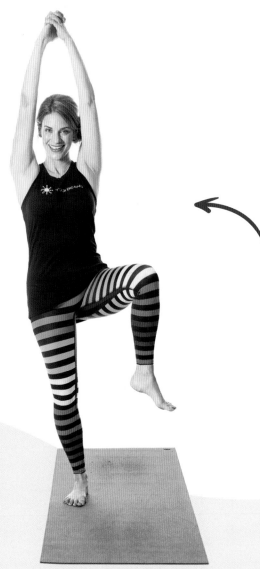

WHO AM I?

I am the **largest** land mammal on **Earth.** I have an **excellent memory** and I am best known for my **large trunk.**

LET'S MOVE!

Stand with your legs hip distance apart. Bring your hands together to form your elephant "trunk." **Swing** your trunk **up, down** and **side to side.** Try taking some **big elephant stomps!**

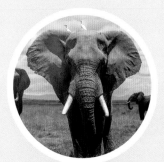

AGE: 2+

POSE TYPE: Standing

ANATOMICAL FOCUS: Arms, Legs

VALUE: I AM united

Rhinoceros

Ardha Uttanasana Variation

WHO AM I?

The name of this animal comes from Greek words that mean **"nose-horn."**

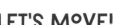

LET'S MOVE!

Keeping your legs straight, bend forward and place your hands on your forehead to **form your rhinoceros horn.** Try and keep your back as **straight** as a line.

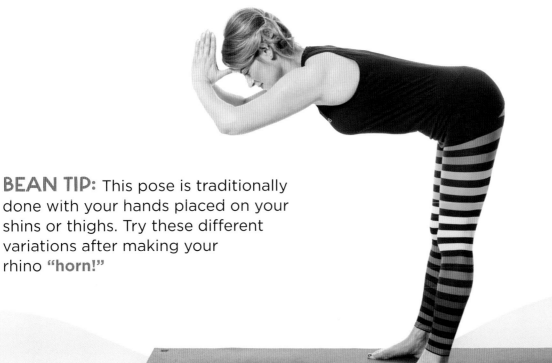

BEAN TIP: This pose is traditionally done with your hands placed on your shins or thighs. Try these different variations after making your rhino **"horn!"**

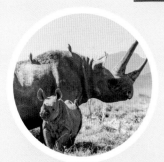

AGE: 3+

POSE TYPE: Standing

ANATOMICAL FOCUS: Legs, Back

VALUE: I AM agile

UNDER THE
SeA

Rub in your **suntan lotion,** grab your **snorkel** and dive into the **deep blue sea** to explore the underwater world below. With these poses we will get to know our **ocean friends!**

During your adventure, if you see any plastic floating around, try and pick it up. We want to keep our oceans clean.

WHICH SEA ANIMAL IS YOUR FAVORITE?

Crab

Purvottanasana Variation

WHO AM I?

I have **pincers** (claws) and I am known for my unique **sideways walk.**

LET'S MOVE!

Sit on the floor with your hands behind you, fingers facing toward your feet. Bend your knees and lift your bottom up off the floor. Crabs walk **side to side.** Say **"hello"** by lifting one of your legs up in the air.

BEAN TIP: To make this pose **extra tricky,** try lifting one arm and one leg at the same time!

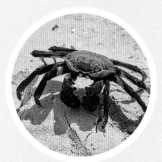

AGE: 2+

POSE TYPE: Backbend, Core

ANATOMICAL FOCUS: Arms, Legs, Core

VALUE: I AM protected

Dolphin

Ardha Pincha Mayurasana

WHO AM I?

I swim in pods with my friends. I am **intelligent** and **playful.**

LET'S MOVE!

Begin on all four limbs and lower down onto your forearms. Now, lift your bottom into Downward Dog pose (page 13) while staying on your forearms. **Gently rock back-and-forth** as if you are a **dolphin riding a wave!**

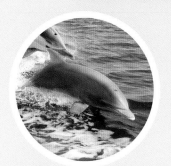

AGE: 5+

POSE TYPE: Inversion

ANATOMICAL FOCUS: Shoulders, Legs

VALUE: I AM friendly

Octopus

Navasana Variation

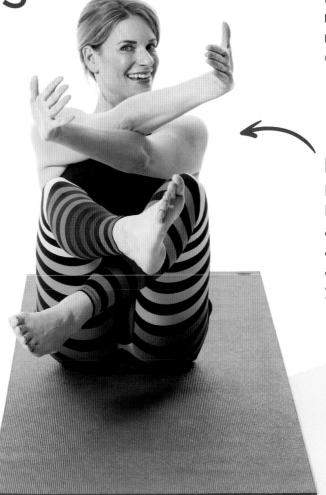

WHO AM I?

I am an **invertebrate,** which means I have **no bones.** I am most recognized by my **eight arms.**

LET'S MOVE!

Begin in Boat pose (page 105). Lift your arms and legs up in the air. **Find your balance!** Wiggle and wave your arms and legs across your body and imagine you have eight arms!

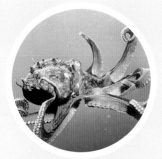

AGE: 3+

POSE TYPE: Core

ANATOMICAL FOCUS: Core

VALUE: I AM flexible

Starfish

Utthita Tadasana

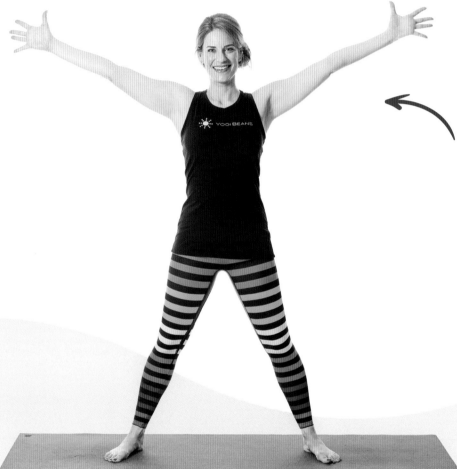

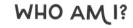

WHO AM I?

I have **five arms.** The word **"fish"** is in my name, but I am actually **not a fish!**

LET'S MOVE!

Begin in Mountain pose (page 19). **Now, burst into Starfish pose!** Take a deep breath right into the center of your belly with your arms reaching out wide.

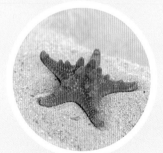

AGE: 2+

POSE TYPE: Standing

ANATOMICAL FOCUS: Arms, Legs

VALUE: I AM self-aware

Turtle

Kurmasana

WHO AM I?

I can live to be **100 years old** and I have a **shell** on my back. I am known for being **slow and steady**.

LET'S MOVE!

Sit with your knees dropped off to the side, and slide your arms underneath your legs. On an inhalation, **pop your head out of your shell** as if you are coming up to the surface for air!

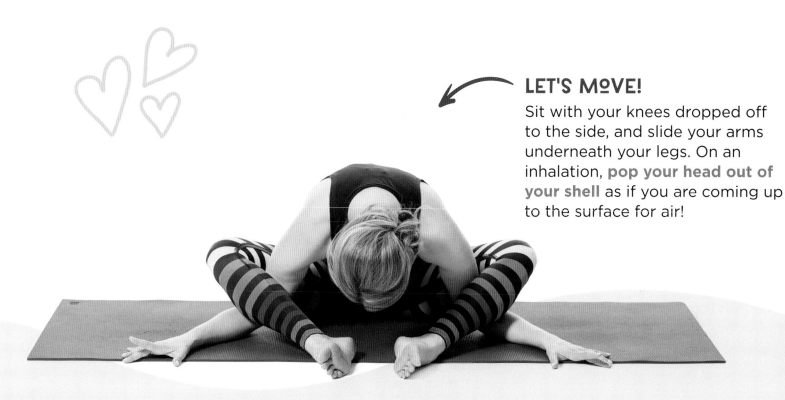

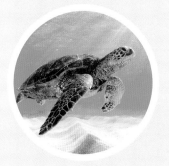

AGE: 5+

POSE TYPE: Forward Bend

ANATOMICAL FOCUS: Legs, Back

VALUE: I AM present

Seahorse

Ardha Matsyendrasana

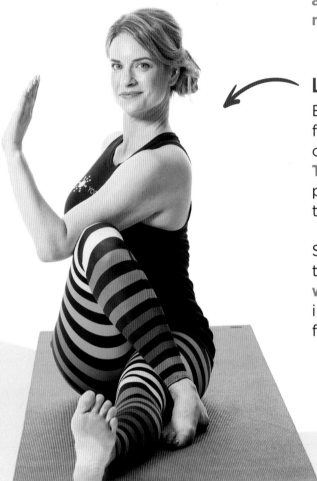

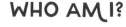

WHO AM I?

The shape of my head **resembles a horse**, which is **how I got my name.**

LET'S MOVE!

Begin with your legs straight in front of you. Bend one knee and cross it over your opposite leg. **Twist** toward your bent knee and place your opposite elbow on the outside.

Seahorses adjust the air inside their bodies to move. **Try to move with your breath** while moving in and out of your twist. Don't forget to switch to the other side!

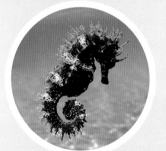

AGE: 5+

POSE TYPE: Twist

ANATOMICAL FOCUS: Back, Legs

VALUE: I AM content

ON THE
NATURe TRAIL

MOTHER EARTH IS AMAZING!

You may have already noticed that many yoga poses get their names from objects found in nature. Lace up those hiking boots and head out to the **nature trail.** We are going to **flap** our colorful **butterfly wings,** learn how to be **strong like a tree,** and **scuttle** along the forest floor like a **little squirrel.** Notice the changes in nature from season to season.

Tree

Vrksasana

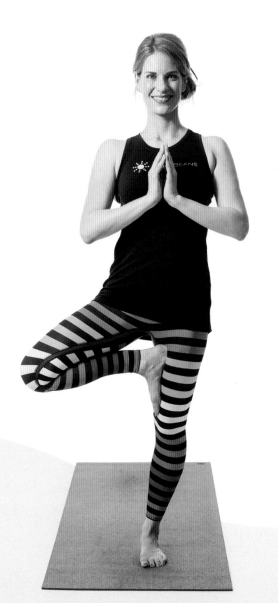

WHAT AM I?

I am made up of roots, a trunk, branches and leaves. My name can be **maple, oak or spruce.**

LET'S MOVE!

Place the sole of your foot onto your opposite ankle or thigh and find your *drishti.* **Move** your arms to create different branches. Remember that trees **sway in the wind,** so if you are wobbling, **it may just be a windy day!**

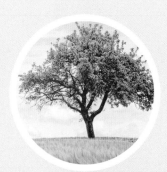

AGE: 2+

POSE TYPE: Balancing

ANATOMICAL FOCUS: Legs

VALUE: I AM rooted

Flower

Vikasitakamalasana

WHAT AM I?

I can be a **rose,** a **tulip** or a **daisy.**
Which is your favorite to **smell?**

LET'S MOVE!

Begin in Butterfly pose (page 50).
Weave your arms underneath
your legs and **lift** your feet off
the floor with your toes touching.
Take a deep breath and **smell the
fragrant flower.**

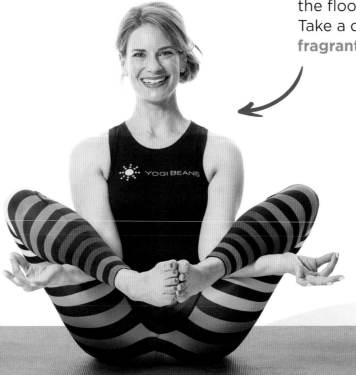

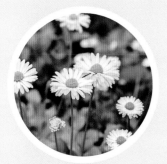

AGE: 3+

ANATOMICAL FOCUS: Core, Legs

POSE TYPE: Seated, Balancing

VALUE: I AM beautiful

Butterfly

Baddha Konasana

WHƏT COLOR iS YOUR BUTTERFLY?

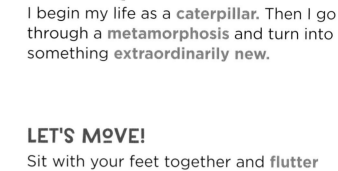

WHO AM I?

I begin my life as a **caterpillar**. Then I go through a **metamorphosis** and turn into something **extraordinarily new**.

LET'S MOVE!

Sit with your feet together and **flutter** your legs (your "wings," that is) fast and slow. Try stretching one wing and then the other.

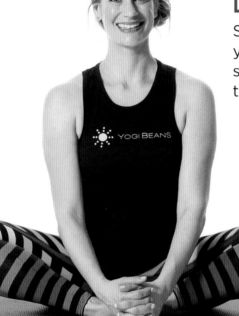

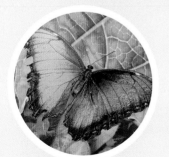

AGE: 2+

POSE TYPE: Seated

ANATOMICAL FOCUS: Legs

VALUE: I AM transformative

Rainbow

Vashistasana

WHAT AM I?

I may appear in the sky after a **rainstorm.** I am made up of seven colors. **Can you name the colors?**

LET'S MOVE!

From Downward Dog pose (page 13), come into Plank pose (page 90). Next, roll onto the outer edge of one foot. Keep one arm **planted** on the ground and **lift** your other arm to the **clouds.** Can you make your body **arc like a rainbow?** To modify, lower one knee down to the floor.

BEAN TIP: Try listing the colors of the rainbow while you hold this pose.

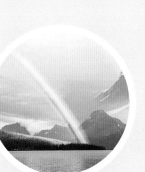

AGE: 5+

POSE TYPE: Arm Balance

ANATOMICAL FOCUS: Core, Legs

VALUE: I AM peaceful

Fly / Firefly

Bhujapidasana / Tittibhasana

LET'S MOVE!

Begin in Frog pose (page 26), and then take your hands underneath your bottom and plant them on the pinky toe sides of your feet. Use your belly muscles to **lift** your feet off the floor into Fly pose. From here, try to **extend** your legs straight to come into Firefly pose and **light up the sky!**

WHO AM I?

If you leave a window open, I may **fly** through and **buzz** around your home.

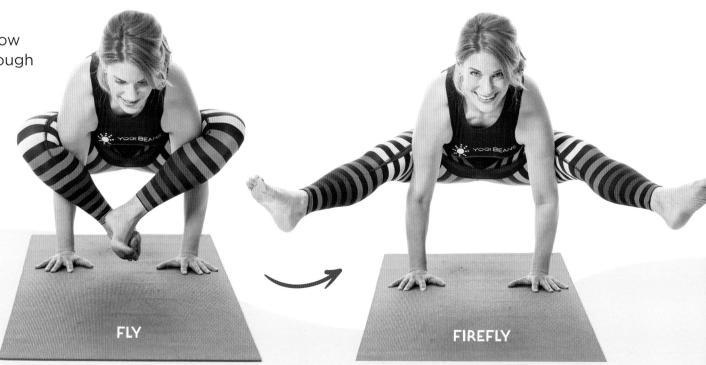

FLY

FIREFLY

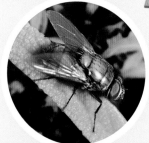

AGE: 8+

POSE TYPE: Arm Balance

ANATOMICAL FOCUS: Core

VALUE: I AM clear

Crawling Bug

Utthita Tittibhasana Variation

I come in all shapes and sizes. I have **millions** of different species that are found all across the world. I am usually **small enough to crawl** on your hand or arm.

LET'S MOVE!

Squat down low and wrap your arms around your legs. Try to **skitter around** as if you are a bug looking for food at a picnic!

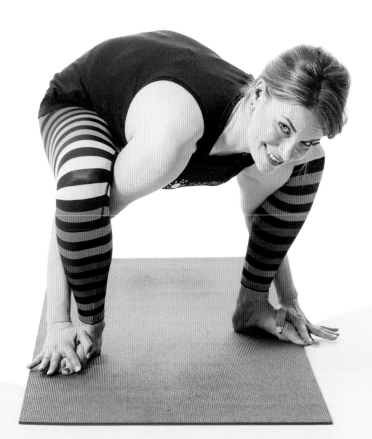

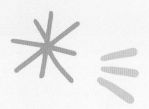

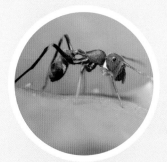

AGE: 8+

POSE TYPE: Forward Bend

ANATOMICAL FOCUS: Back, Legs

VALUE: I AM diligent

Squirrel

Salabhasana Variation

WHO AM I?

I have a **bushy tail** and great climbing skills. **Acorns** are my favorite treat.

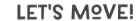

LET'S MOVE!

Begin by lying on your belly. **Steady your squirrel** by placing the palms of your hands underneath your hips. Create your squirrel's **bushy tail** by lifting one leg straight behind you; you can help hold it up by bending your other leg.

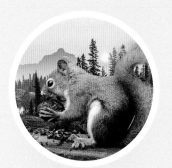

AGE: 8+

POSE TYPE: Backbend

ANATOMICAL FOCUS: Back, Legs

VALUE: I AM resourceful

Waterfall

Paschimottanasana

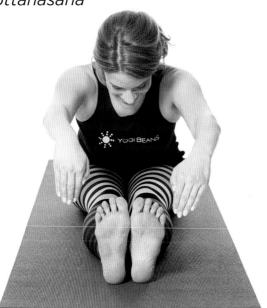

WHAT AM I?

I can be found at the top of a mountain. I **cascade my way down** the mountain into a pool of **water.**

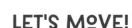

LET'S MOVE!

With your legs straight in front of you, inhale as you reach your arms up. Exhale as the water falls over your toes. **Let out a big whoosh!** For a deep stretch, hold onto your feet and take a few breaths. Imagine the waterfall is **flowing over you.**

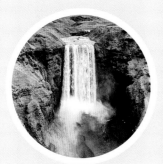

AGE: 3+

POSE TYPE: Forward Bend

ANATOMICAL FOCUS: Legs, Back

VALUE: I AM open

Lotus

Padmasana

WHAT AM I?

This **special flower** grows in the mud and reminds us that **beauty** can come from dark places.

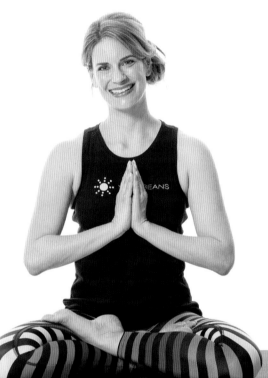

LET'S MOVE!

Begin sitting with your legs extended. Bend one knee and bring your ankle to your opposite hip crease with the sole of your foot facing upward. Now, bend the other knee and cross it over to the other hip crease. **This pose requires flexibility in the hips.** If it feels uncomfortable, first try practicing this pose with only one leg bent (known as Half Lotus pose).

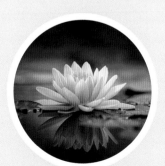

AGE: 5+

POSE TYPE: Seated

ANATOMICAL FOCUS: Hips

VALUE: I AM pure

BLAST OFF TO
OUTER SPACE

Step into your **spacesuit** and put on your **astronaut helmet**.
It is time to **blast off** into outer space! Travel through
unknown galaxies, whizz by **stars** and maybe
even land on the **moon.**

3-2-1, BLAST OFF!

Alien

Utkata Konasana Variation

WHO AM I?

I live on a **planet** other than **Earth**. I am also called an **extraterrestrial**.

LET'S MOVE!

Stand in a slight squat with your arms out wide and bent at a 90-degree angle. As you **open and close** your arms and legs, imagine what **silly sounds and faces** your alien makes!

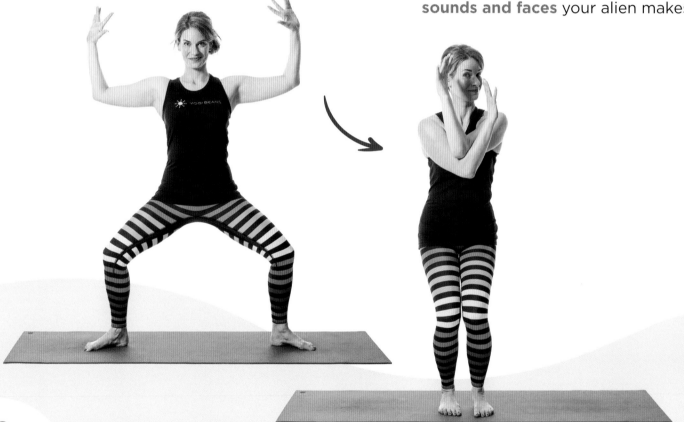

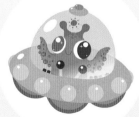

AGE: 3+

POSE TYPE: Standing

ANATOMICAL FOCUS: Legs

VALUE: I AM unique

Rocket Ship

Utkatasana Variation

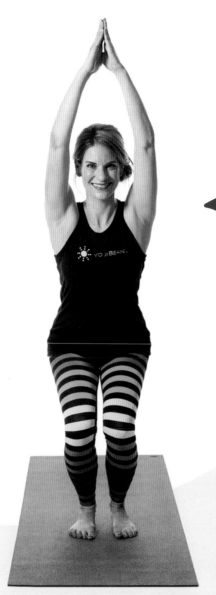

WHAT AM I?

I am what an **astronaut** rides to **blast off** into outer space.

LET'S MOVE!

Standing with your feet together, bend your knees and point your arms up to the stars. **3-2-1, blast off!** Run around your mat to lift off into outer space.

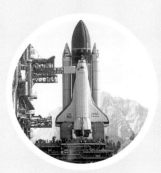

AGE: 2+

POSE TYPE: Standing

ANATOMICAL FOCUS: Legs

VALUE: I AM motivated

Star

Utthita Tadasana

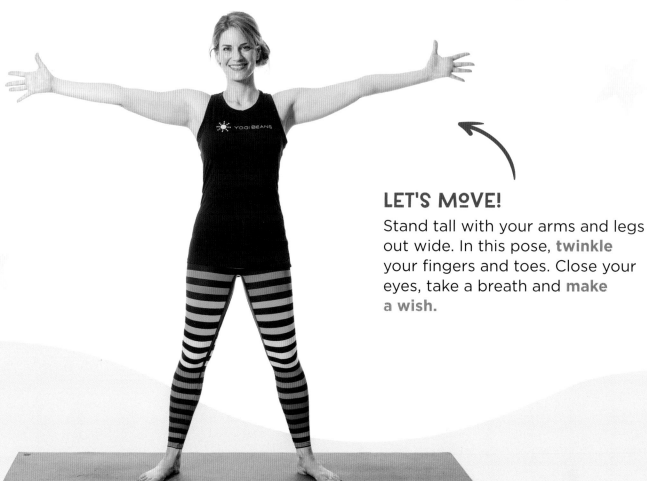

I **twinkle** in the night sky.

LET'S MOVE!

Stand tall with your arms and legs out wide. In this pose, **twinkle** your fingers and toes. Close your eyes, take a breath and **make a wish.**

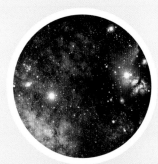

AGE: 2+

POSE TYPE: Standing

ANATOMICAL FOCUS: Arms, Legs

VALUE: I AM authentic

Half Moon

Ardha Chandrasana

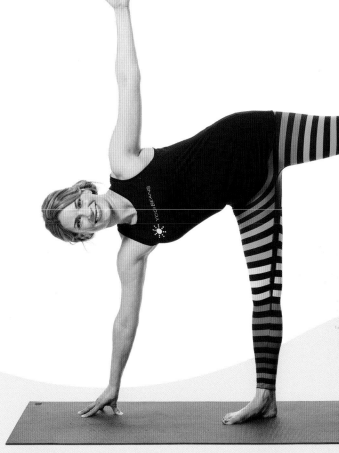

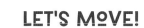

LET'S MOVE!

Begin in Star pose (page 60). Slowly tip over as if **you are a falling star.** Reach your back leg up into the air. Can you hold this pose for **three breaths?**

AGE: 5+

POSE TYPE: Balancing

ANATOMICAL FOCUS: Legs

VALUE: I AM intuitive

Sun Breath

Surya Namaskar Variation

WHAT AM I?

I am the **star** at the center of our **Solar System.**

LET'S MOVE!

Inhale and reach your arms up to **"catch the sun."** Exhale and bend forward to **"let it go."**

BEAN TIP: This pose is a great introduction to linking breath with movement.

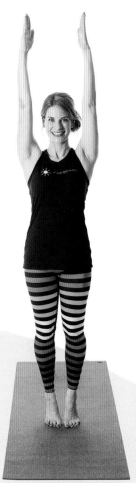

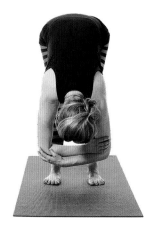

AGE: 2+

POSE TYPE: Standing

ANATOMICAL FOCUS: Arms, Legs

VALUE: I AM powerful

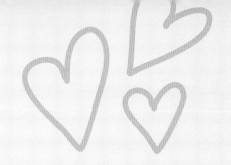

PEOPLE
POSES

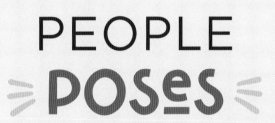

Have you ever wondered what it feels like to **skydive, wrangle** a bull, **dance** on a Broadway stage or be as **brave** as a warrior? Every human being is **special and unique.** Try on a few different poses to discover how it feels to move your body like different people.

Warrior

Virabhadrasana Variations

WHO AM I?

I am **brave** and **courageous!** I protect people and stand up for **justice!**

LET'S MOVE!

Use positive "I AM" *mantras* as you flow through each warrior variation:

I AM a **Strong** Warrior: Warrior 1
I AM a **Proud** Warrior: Warrior 2
I AM a **Peaceful** Warrior: Reverse Warrior
I AM a **Flying** Warrior: Warrior 3

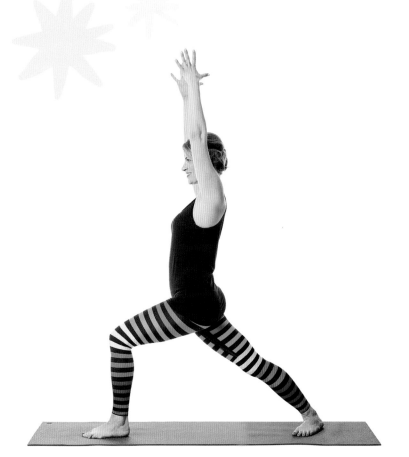

STRONG

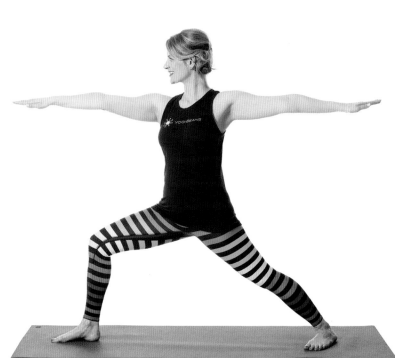

PROUD

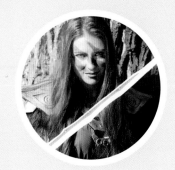

AGE: 5+

POSE TYPE: Standing, Balancing

ANATOMICAL FOCUS: Legs

VALUE: I AM protective

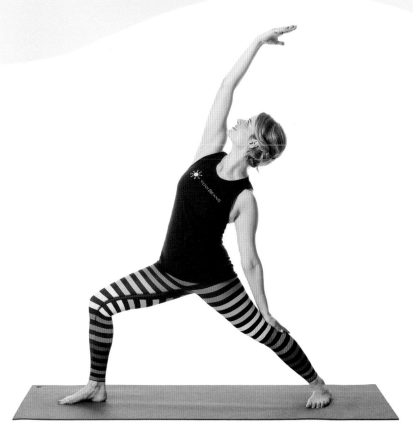

PEACEFUL

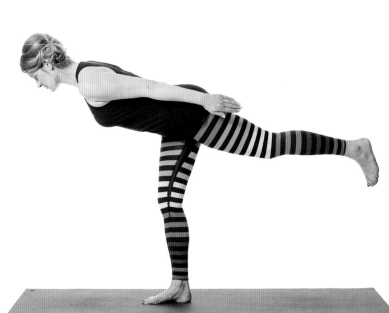

FLYING

Dancer

Natarajasana

WHO AM I?

I am a performer who loves to move. I may practice **ballet, tap** or **hip-hop.**

LET'S MOVE!

Begin in Mountain pose (page 19). Focus your gaze on something that is still and find your ***drishti.*** Now, try to **float** your leg up off the floor behind you. **Bend** your knee and hold onto your foot if you can reach it. Can you find **balance** in this pose?

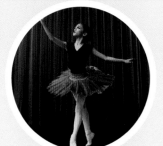

AGE: 5+

POSE TYPE: Balancing

ANATOMICAL FOCUS: Legs, Back

VALUE: I AM graceful

Guitar Player

WHO AM I?

I play a **string instrument** that I can **pluck** or **strum** to make music.

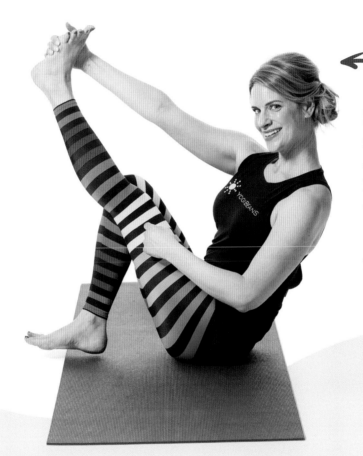

LET'S MOVE!

Start sitting with your knees bent and extend one leg up high. Grab your "guitar" with your opposite arm and **strum the strings.** Let's play some rock-n-roll by rolling back and forth! **What song are you strumming along to?**

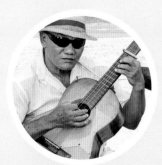

AGE: 5+

POSE TYPE: Seated

ANATOMICAL FOCUS: Legs

VALUE: I AM Expressive

Skydiver

Shalambasana Variation

WHO AM I?

I wear a **parachute** and **jump** out of planes for a **thrill.**

LET'S MOVE!

Start by lying on your belly. Imagine you just jumped out of a plane and lift your arms with bent elbows and your legs too. **Feel your breath move like the wind** as you descend to the ground. All the buildings and cars below look **so small!**

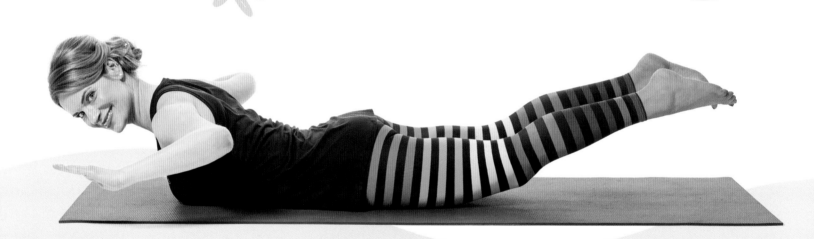

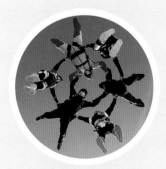

AGE: 3+

POSE TYPE: Backbend

ANATOMICAL FOCUS: Back, Shoulders

VALUE: I AM expansive

Lumberjack

Kashtha Takshanasana

WHO AM I?

I cut down **trees** for **wood**.
I am also known as a **logger**.

BEAN TIP: This is a great pose to **release energy or frustration** when you need to calm down.

Inhale as you reach your arms up. On your exhalation say, **"HA!"** and **swing your arms down** as if you are chopping wood.

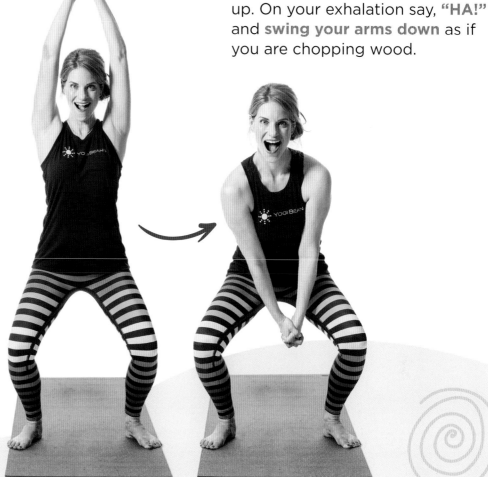

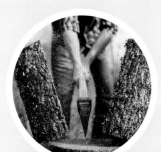

AGE: 3+

POSE TYPE: Standing

ANATOMICAL FOCUS: Legs, Arms

VALUE: I AM intentional

Cowboy / Cowgirl

Utkata Konasana Variation

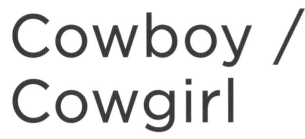

WHO AM I?

I ride a horse and tend cattle on a **ranch.** I might greet you by saying, **"Howdy, partner!"**

LET'S MOVE!

Sit on your horse and get ready to ride. **Swing your lasso** round-and-round and say, **"Yeehaw!"**

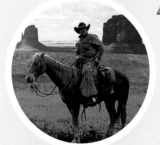

AGE: 2+

POSE TYPE: Standing

ANATOMICAL FOCUS: Legs

VALUE: I AM self-disciplined

Happy Baby

Ananda Balasana

WHO AM I?

I wear a **diaper** and sleep in a **crib**. I am happy, although I **cry** when I am hungry, wet or tired.

LET'S MOVE!

Lie on your back and bring your knees in toward your chest. Reach for your toes. **Rock side to side** like a happy baby giggling in their crib.

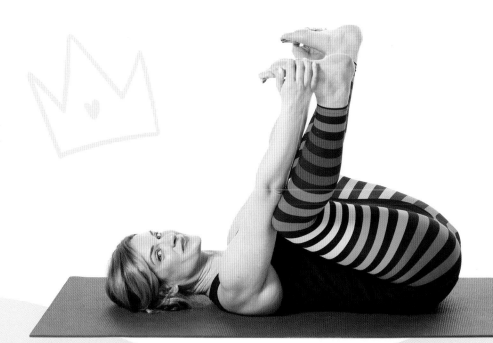

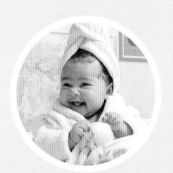

AGE: 2+

POSE TYPE: Hip Opening

ANATOMICAL FOCUS: Hips

VALUES: I AM love

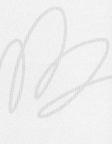

Scuba Diver

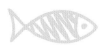

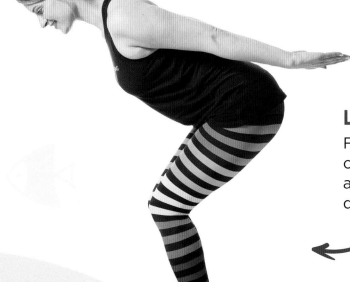

WHO AM I?

I use special equipment to breathe underwater and explore **reefs, marine animals, caves** and **shipwrecks!**

LET'S MOVE!

From Chair pose (page 115), stand on your tiptoes and reach your arms behind you. Imagine you are diving into the **big blue sea.**

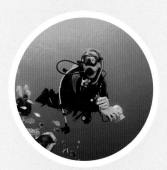

AGE: 3+

POSE TYPE: Standing

ANATOMICAL FOCUS: Legs

VALUE: I AM agile

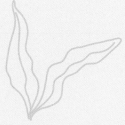

BIRD
WORLD

It is time to **spread your wings** and **soar into the sky!** In this chapter, you will become small birds, fast birds and birds that can stand on just one leg. Fly above the horizon and **see how high you can fly!**

Flamingo

WHO AM I?

I am born with **gray feathers,** which **turn to pink** because of the type of food I eat.

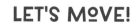

LET'S MOVE!

From Mountain pose (page 19), extend your arms out to the sides. Float one leg up in the air and **balance** like a **resting flamingo.**

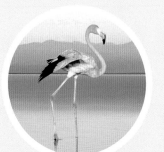

AGE: 3+

POSE TYPE: Balancing

ANATOMICAL FOCUS: Legs, Core

VALUE: I AM vibrant

Bird on a Branch

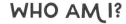

WHO AM I?

I am a bird who loves to **perch** on these sturdy **limbs** that grow from trees.

LET'S MOVE!

Stand on your tiptoes in Mountain pose (page 19) and slowly lower down to a kneeling position. **Flap your "wings" up and down** as you balance on your tiptoes.

BEAN TIP: For added fun, try looking up and down and side to side. **Let out a "tweet, tweet!"** to say hello to your bird friends on other branches!

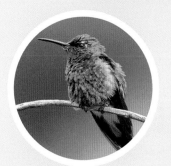

AGE: 3+

POSE TYPE: Balancing

ANATOMICAL FOCUS: Core

VALUE: I AM balanced

Crow

Bakasana

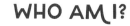

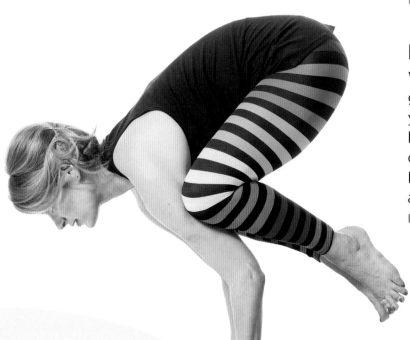

WHO AM I?

I am **extremely intelligent** and known for my loud **caw** and shiny **black feathers.**

LET'S MOVE!

With your hands flat on the ground, create a "shelf" with your arms and place your elbows high on the shelf. Try and **lift** one foot at a time to take flight. Remember the Yogi Beans affirmation: **It is a Yoga Practice, not a Yoga Perfect!**

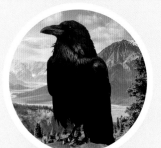

AGE: 5+

POSE TYPE: Core

ANATOMICAL FOCUS: Arms, Core

VALUE: I AM intelligent

Eagle

Garudasana

BEAN TIP: Simplify this pose by crossing your arms over your chest and keeping both feet on the floor with one leg in front of the other.

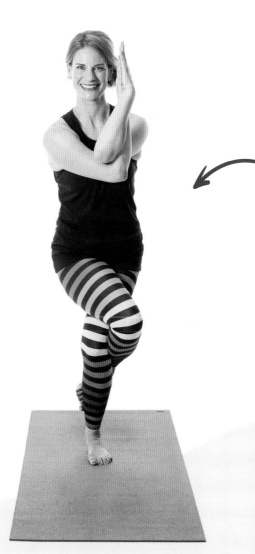

WHO AM I?

I am the **national bird** of the United States. I can be found on a **one-dollar bill** or a **quarter.**

LET'S MOVE!

Standing with your feet together, wrap one leg around the other and do the same with your arms. Gently bend your knee to lower down a little. Turn on your **eagle eyes** and **steady your gaze** to find balance. Make sure to switch sides.

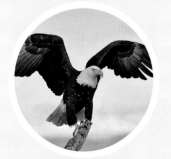

AGE: 3+

POSE TYPE: Balancing

ANATOMICAL FOCUS: Shoulders, Legs

VALUE: I AM focused

Albatross

Dandayamana Bharmanasana Variation

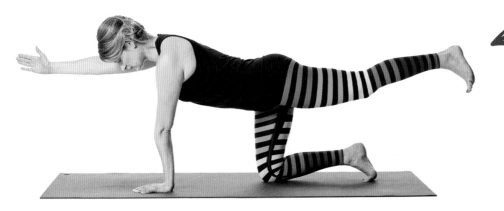

WHO AM I?

I have the **longest wingspan** of any living bird.

LET'S MOVE!

Starting on your hands and knees, extend one arm (wing) and opposite leg. Once steady, open your arm and leg out to the side. **See how long you can balance and soar!** Don't forget to switch sides to fly with your other wing!

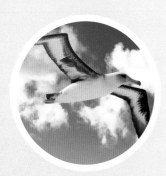

AGE: 5+

POSE TYPE: Core

ANATOMICAL FOCUS: Arms, Legs

VALUE: I AM free

Peacock

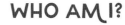

WHO AM I?

I am loved for my beautiful fan of **blue** and **green tail feathers.**

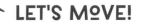

LET'S MOVE!

Lying on your back, show off your peacock feathers by opening and closing your legs and arms. Play around with moving **super fast** and then **super slow.**

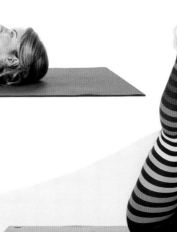

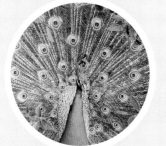

AGE: 2+

POSE TYPE: Hip Opening

ANATOMICAL FOCUS: Core, Legs

VALUE: I AM respectful

Owl

Vajrasana Variation

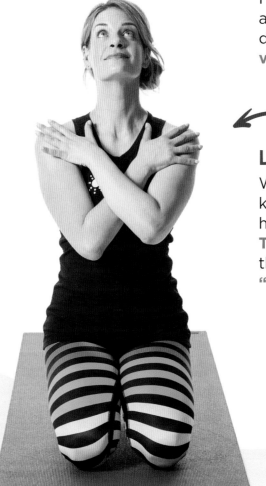

WHO AM I?

I am nocturnal, which means I am active at **night** and I sleep during the **day.** People say I am **very wise.**

BEAN TIP: To make this pose trickier, try balancing on your toes while shifting your gaze.

LET'S MOVE!

While sitting quietly on your knees, cross your arms over your heart and focus your gaze up. **Turn** your head side to side and then up and down. Let out a slow **"hoot, hoot."**

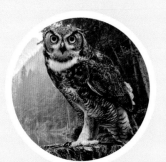

AGE: 3+

POSE TYPE: Seated

ANATOMICAL FOCUS: Neck

VALUE: I AM mindful

Pigeon

Eka Pada Rajakapotasana

WHO AM I?

You can find me in crowded city **parks** or hanging out on the **windowsill** of a building.

LET'S MOVE!

From a seated position, bend one knee with your foot close to your body. Extend the opposite leg behind you. **This pigeon is tired!** Be a sleeping pigeon and lower your head down to the floor (or as far down as you can).

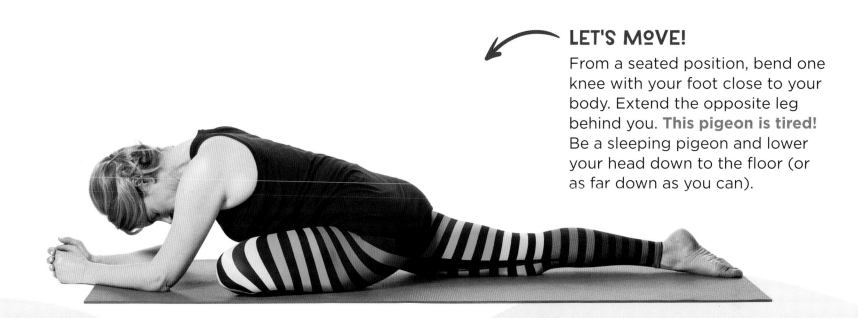

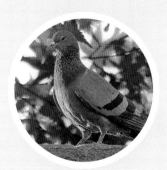

AGE: 5+

POSE TYPE: Hip Opening

ANATOMICAL FOCUS: Hips

VALUE: I AM social

Ostrich

Parivrtta Anjaneyasana

WHO AM I?

I do not fly, but my **long legs** help me to **run** very **fast!**

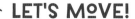

LET'S MOVE!

Start in a standing lunge and lower one arm to the ground. Stretch your other arm to the sky and imagine it is your long ostrich neck. Then, slowly lower your arm back down as if you are **burying your ostrich head in the sand.** Switch sides and repeat.

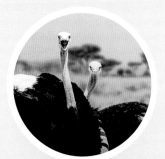

AGE: 5+

POSE TYPE: Twist

ANATOMICAL FOCUS: Legs, Shoulders

VALUE: I AM honest

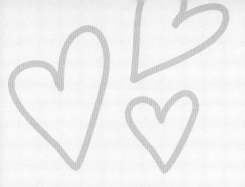

FANTASY
ADVENTURe

Invite your imagination to go wild and fill your mind with wonder, as you journey through a land of **fantastical adventure**. From a strong and fierce **dinosaur** to a beautiful **mermaid** and even a silly **monster,** there are so many **fun creatures** to meet in this chapter!

REMEMBER, MAGIC CAN BE FOUND ALL AROUND YOU AS LONG AS YOU BELIEVE!

Unicorn

Anjaneyasana

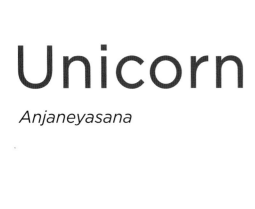

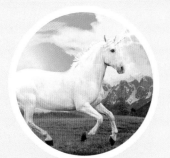

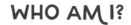

WHO AM I?

I am a **magical creature** that looks like a **horse.** I have a special horn on my head that makes me **unique.**

LET'S MOVE!

Begin in a low lunge with your back knee down. Reach your unicorn horn up to the sky, **shine your heart** and then rise up to gallop around your mat.

AGE: 3+

POSE TYPE: Standing

ANATOMICAL FOCUS: Legs

VALUE: I AM creative

Dinosaur

Padangusthasana

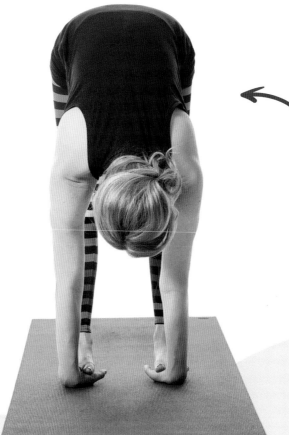

WHO AM I?

My name means **"terrible lizard."** I stomped on this earth over **65 million** years ago.

LET'S MOVE!

Stand on your hands and try taking a few dinosaur **stomps** forward and backward. For added fun, try lifting one leg out to the side and see if you can balance.

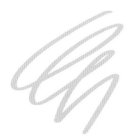

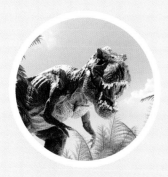

AGE: 3+

POSE TYPE: Forward Bend

ANATOMICAL FOCUS: Legs

VALUE: I AM strong

Mermaid

WHO AM I?

I am a **magical** and **legendary** creature. I have the upper body of a **human** and a **fish** tail instead of legs.

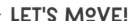

LET'S MOVE!

Sit with your legs bent to one side. With one hand on your foot, reach your other arm up high in the sky as if to touch a shooting star. **Swoosh your mermaid legs** to the opposite side and repeat.

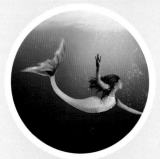

AGE: 3+

POSE TYPE: Seated

ANATOMICAL FOCUS: Core, Legs

VALUE: I AM imaginative

Silly Monster

Utkata Konasana Variation

Some kids are afraid I am hiding under their bed. I promise, **I just want to play!**

LET'S MOVE!

In a wide-legged squat, bring your arms together like in Eagle pose (page 77) and inhale deeply. As you exhale, **stick out** your tongue, **stomp** your feet and **do a silly monster dance!**

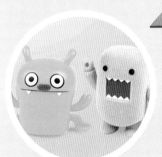

AGE: 3+

POSE TYPE: Standing

ANATOMICAL FOCUS: Legs, Shoulders

VALUE: I AM nonjudgmental

Superyogi

Shalambasana Variation

WHO AM I?

I am not a bird. I am not a plane.
I AM _____ !

LET'S MOVE!

1-2-3 let's soar! Start lying on your belly. Lift your arms and legs off the floor with one arm straight in front of you and imagine you are flying over your city or town. Lower back down and **take flight again,** this time with the other arm in front.

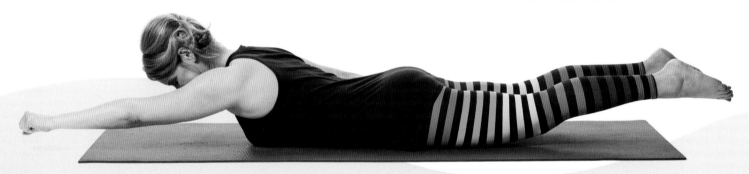

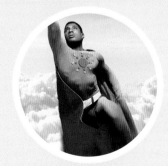

AGE: 3+

POSE TYPE: Backbend

ANATOMICAL FOCUS: Back, Core

VALUE: I AM motivational

Sea Serpent

Anantasana

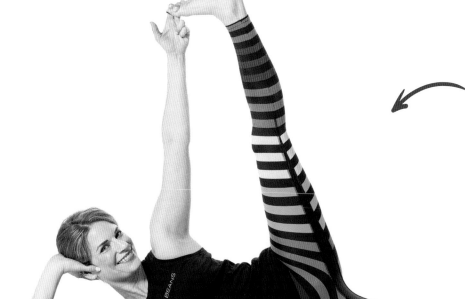

WHO AM I?

I am a mythical and legendary **sea creature** that looks like a long **snake.**

LET'S MOVE!

Begin lying on your side. Reach for your toes or use a strap or towel to wrap around your foot. Slowly **extend your leg** up toward the ceiling as if you are a sea serpent **sticking your head out** of the murky waters.

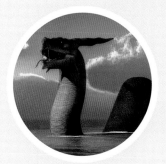

AGE: 5+

POSE TYPE: Hip Opening

ANATOMICAL FOCUS: Legs, Core

VALUE: I AM protective

Pirate's Plank

Phalakasana

WHO AM I?

Ahoy matey! Don't make me angry or I will make you walk the plank!

LET'S MOVE!

Begin in Downward Dog pose (page 13). Roll forward so your shoulders are over your wrists. Imagine a balloon is pulling your belly button up so your muscles are engaged and your back is straight. How many breaths you can take while holding this pose is the number of steps you take as you **walk the pirate's plank!**

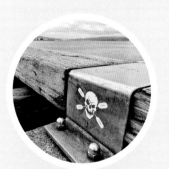

AGE: 5+

POSE TYPE: Core

ANATOMICAL FOCUS: Core

VALUE: I AM solid

POLAR
EXPRESS

Grab your hat and gloves—we're going to the **Arctic!** Among
the **snow-covered mountain peaks** and narrow water valleys
called **fjords** (FEE-yords), you'll learn about the **strong** and
resilient animals that survive here in some of the **harshest**
of wintry conditions.

Snowball

LET'S MOVE!

Sit on the floor and **hug** your knees into your chest. **Roll** back and forth to make a snowball. For a challenge, try to roll and stand without using your hands!

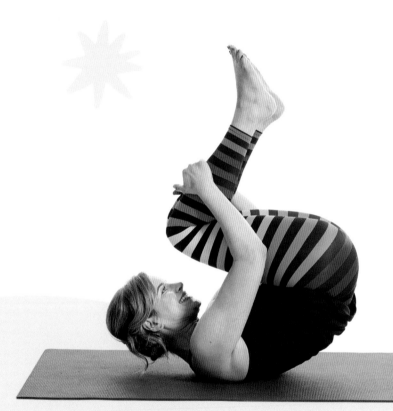

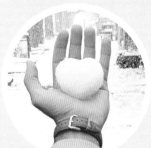

AGE: 3+

POSE TYPE: Seated

ANATOMICAL FOCUS: Core

VALUE: I AM energy

Polar Bear

WHO AM I?

My skin is **black** underneath my **white fur!** This allows me to absorb more sunlight to keep me **warm.**

LET'S MOVE!

From Downward Dog pose (page 13), begin to take a few polar bear walks off your mat while staying on your toes. Imagine you are walking on a sheet of ice. **Watch out—it is slippery!**

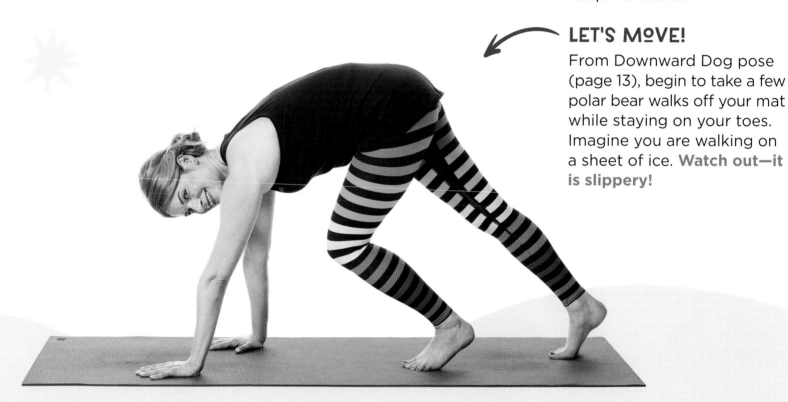

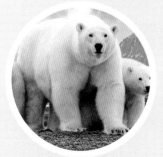

AGE: 2+

POSE TYPE: Inversion

ANATOMICAL FOCUS: Arms, Legs

VALUE: I AM patient

Seal

Begin in Mouse pose (page 17).

WHO AM I?

I have a slick **fur coat** that helps me **glide** through the water.
I bark, too!

LET'S MOVE!

Begin in Mouse pose (page 17). As you inhale, **stretch** your arms up in the air. On your exhale, lower both arms down. **"Seal barking" is encouraged!**

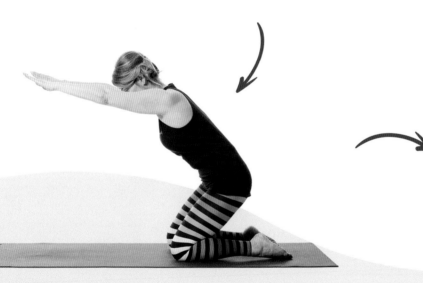

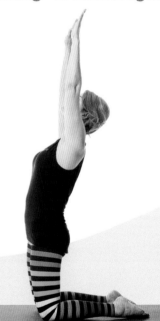

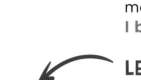

AGE: 2+

POSE TYPE: Seated

ANATOMICAL FOCUS: Core, Back

VALUE: I AM happy

Whale

Shalambasana Variation

WHO AM I?

I am the **largest animal** on our **planet.** I come to the surface of the ocean to breathe through a blowhole at the top of my head.

LET'S MOVE!

Lie flat on your belly. Breathe in and interlace your hands together behind your back. On your inhale, **lift your legs and chest up** and imagine you are coming to the surface to **take a breath.**

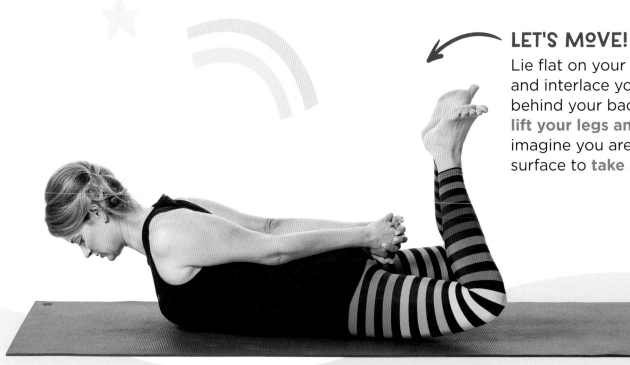

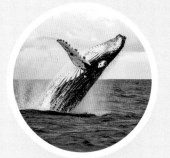

AGE: 5+

POSE TYPE: Backbend

ANATOMICAL FOCUS: Back, Shoulders, Legs

VALUE: I AM communicative

Penguin

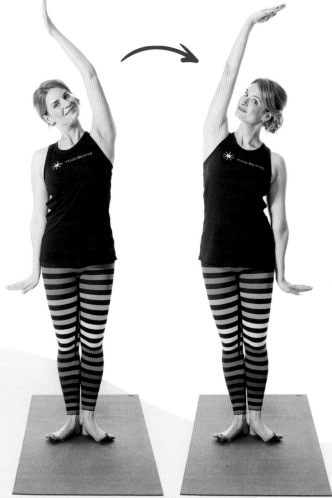

WHO AM I?

I am a bird who lives in **cold climates.** My fur is black and white. Does it look like I wear a **tuxedo?**

LET'S MOVE!

Stand with your heels together and toes apart. Keep this stance as you stretch from side to side. **Waddling is optional!**

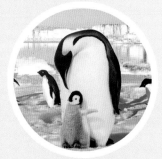

AGE: 2+

POSE TYPE: Standing

ANATOMICAL FOCUS: Arms, Legs

VALUE: I AM adaptable

DEEP IN THE
DESERT

Get ready to roll down **sand dunes** and explore **ancient ruins.** On our **desert journey** we will meet the animals and plants that call this arid land their home. Remember to pack your water bottle—**it is hot!**

Camel

Ustrasana

WHO AM I?

WHO AM I?

I am known for the **hump** on my back. I can go **days** without eating food or drinking water.

BEAN TIP: If it feels good, untuck your toes and keep your feet flat for a deeper backbend.

LET'S MOVE!

Stand on your knees with your toes tucked, and place your hands on your lower back for support. Slowly **lean** back and slide your arms down to your heels. Keep your gaze on the bright desert sky above. **Your belly is your camel hump!**

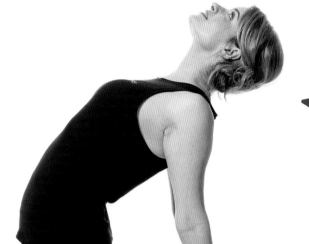

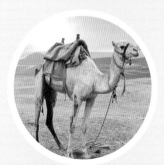

AGE: 5+

POSE TYPE: Backbend

ANATOMICAL FOCUS: Chest, Back

VALUE: I AM resilient

Cactus

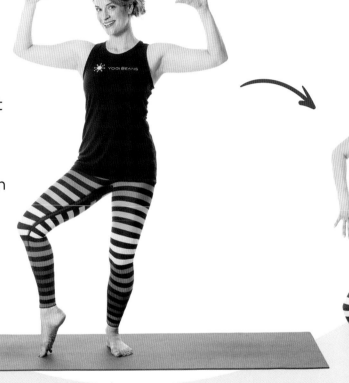

WHAT AM I?

I am a unique plant that lives in **hot** and **dry** climates. I am **prickly** on the outside and **soft** on the inside.

LET'S MOVE!

Begin in Mountain pose (page 19). Start with your arms bent at the elbows to look like a cactus. Do the **"cactus dance"** by moving your **"spikes"** (arms and legs) in different positions and shapes!

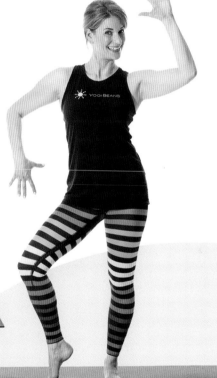

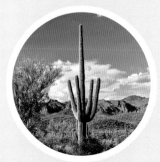

AGE: 2+

POSE TYPE: Standing

ANATOMICAL FOCUS: Legs, Arms

VALUE: I AM persistent

Pyramid

Parsvottanasana

LET'S MOVE!

Begin in Mountain pose (page 19). Next, step one foot forward. Imagine your hips are the headlights of a car and keep them facing forward as you fold over your legs. Notice the **triangle** shape that your legs make.

WHAT AM I?

You can find me in **Egypt.** I am one of the **Seven Wonders** of the Ancient World.

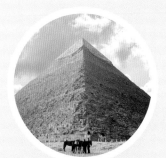

AGE: 3+

POSE TYPE: Forward Bend

ANATOMICAL FOCUS: Legs, Back

VALUE: I AM stable

Lizard

Utthan Pristhasana

WHO AM I?

I am a reptile known for my **dry** and **scaly skin.** Many of us can change color to camouflage with our environment.

LET'S MOVE!

Begin in a low lunge with your back knee down. Place both hands on the inside of your front foot. If you feel steady, try lowering onto your forearms. Stick out your tongue like a lizard and try to to **catch some flies for lunch!**

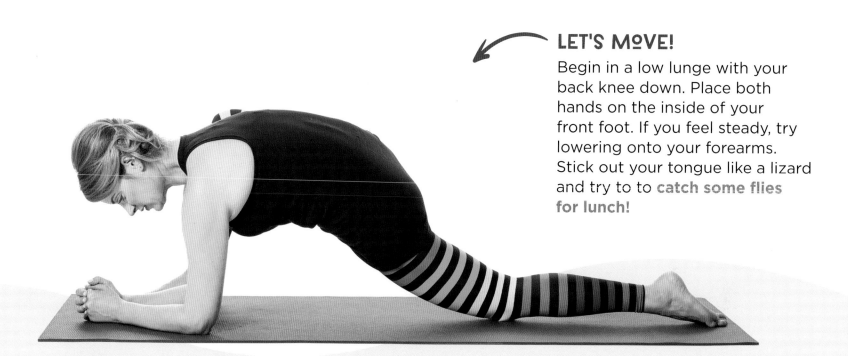

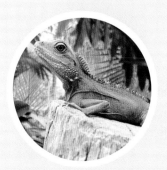

AGE: 5+

POSE TYPE: Hip Opening

ANATOMICAL FOCUS: Legs

VALUE: I AM transformative

Sphinx

Salamba Bhujangasana

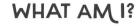

WHAT AM I?

I have the head of a **Pharaoh** and the body of a **lion.** It has been said that in order to pass through me, you must answer a riddle.

LET'S MOVE!

With your elbows fixed to the floor, keep your heart open and lifted in this pose. **Do you know a riddle to say while holding this pose?**

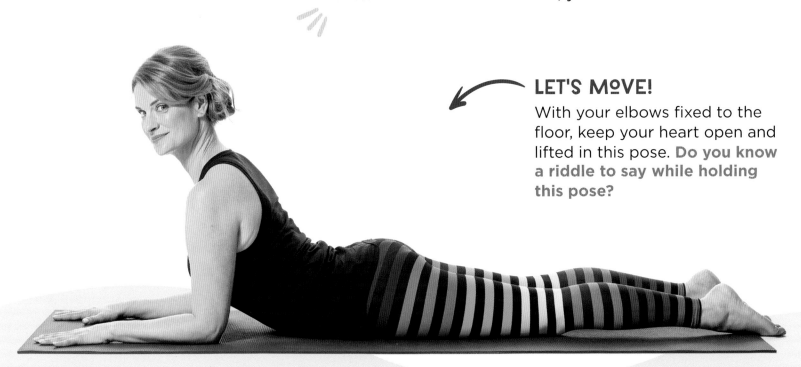

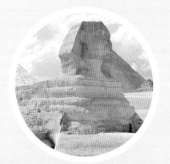

AGE: 2+

POSE TYPE: Backbend

ANATOMICAL FOCUS: Chest, Back

VALUE: I AM introspective

START YOUR
ENGINES

ON YOUR MARK, GET SET, GO!

Whether it is on a **plane, boat** or in a **car,** we will move our bodies to get to where we need to go!

Airplane

Virabradasana III

WHAT AM I?

I am made up of **jet engines, propellers** and **wings.** You can use me to travel long distances, including over oceans.

LET'S MOVE!

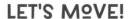

It is time for takeoff! From a standing position, tip forward and raise one leg behind you. Extend your **"wings"** to the sides as you fly through the clouds! Remember to take a **"connecting flight"** and switch sides.

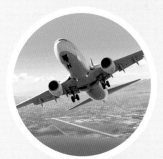

AGE: 3+

POSE TYPE: Balancing

ANATOMICAL FOCUS: Core, Legs

VALUE: I AM focused

Boat

Navasana

WHAT AM I?

I **float** on water. People can ride on me to explore a **lake, river or ocean.**

LET'S MOVE!

Balance on your bottom and slowly lift your chest, legs and arms up high. **Imagine you are raising your sails** on a voyage out to sea. To modify, bend your knees.

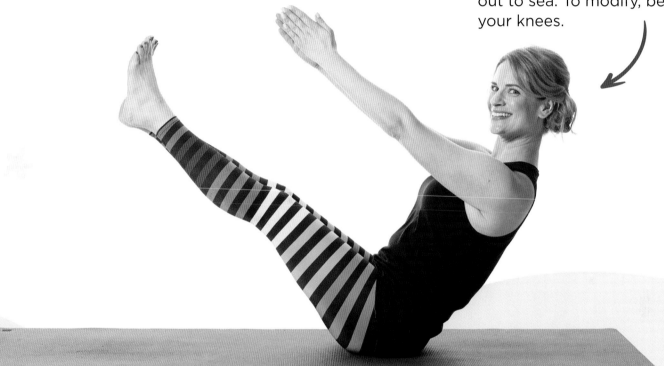

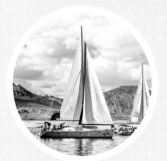

AGE: 2+

POSE TYPE: Core

ANATOMICAL FOCUS: Core

VALUE: I AM steady

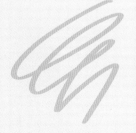

Sleigh

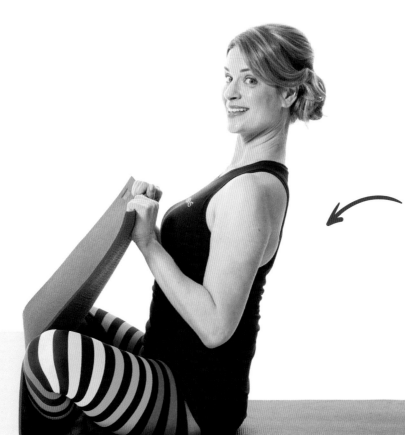

LET'S MOVE!

Sit cross-legged and pick up the edge of your mat. **Roll** back-and-forth as if you are **sledding** down a **snowy mountain.**

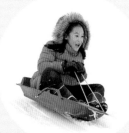

AGE: 2+

POSE TYPE: Seated

ANATOMICAL FOCUS: Core

VALUE: I AM playful

Bicycle

WHAT AM I?

I have two **wheels** and a person must **pedal** to move me.

LET'S MOVE!

Cycle your legs **slowly** as you move up a hill; move your legs **fast** to speed down the hill.

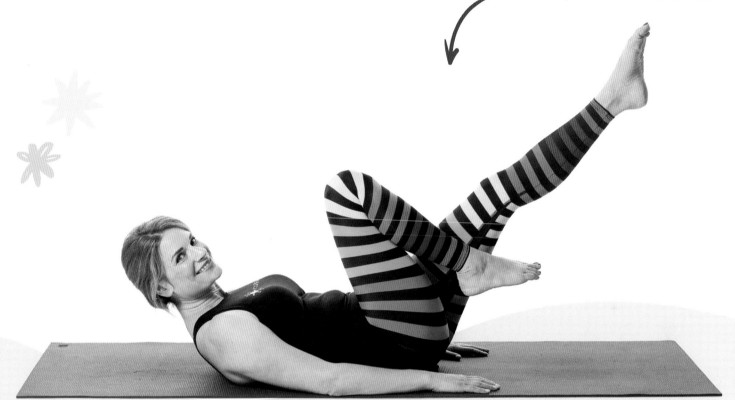

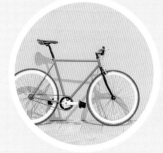

AGE: 2+

POSE TYPE: Core

ANATOMICAL FOCUS: Legs, Core

VALUE: I AM movement

Car

Dandasana

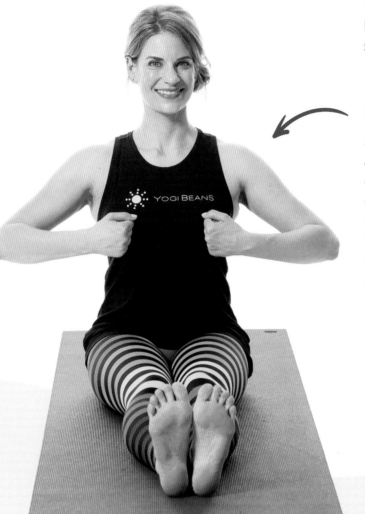

BEAN TIP: On green lights, you can move fast. Be sure to stop when the light turns red!

WHAT AM I?

I have an **engine, four wheels,** a **steering wheel** and **brakes.**

LET'S MOVE!

Sit up tall with a straight back and buckle up! Keep your hands on the steering wheel and **bend** one knee at a time as you use your legs to scooch yourself forward to move your car. Let your engines **"vroom"** and let's get going!

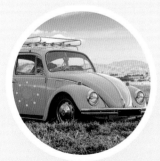

AGE: 2+

POSE TYPE: Seated

ANATOMICAL FOCUS: Legs, Back

VALUE: I AM freedom

Motorcycle

Supta Gomukhasana

WHAT AM I?

I have two **wheels** and I am powered by a **motor.** I love to move **fast!**

LET'S MOVE!

Lying flat on your back, cross one knee on top of the other. Reach for your ankles to feel this stretch. **Steer** your motorcycle by gently **rolling side to side.**

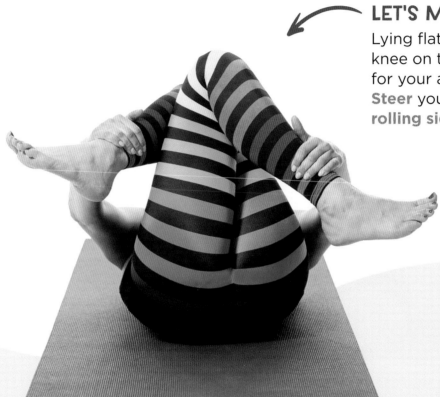

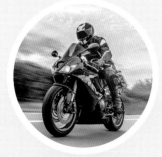

AGE: 5+

POSE TYPE: Hip Opening

ANATOMICAL FOCUS: Hips

VALUE: I AM supported

Bridge

Setu Bandha Sarvangasana

WHAT AM I?

Boats **pass** under me and cars **drive** over me.

LET'S MOVE!

Start on your back with your knees bent. Imagine there is a **balloon** attached to your **heart** as you lift your bottom and bring your chest up to your chin. Clasp your hands under your back as if they are **a little boat** passing under your bridge!

BEAN TIP: This is a good pose to practice before trying Wheel pose on the next page, which is a deeper backbend.

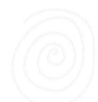

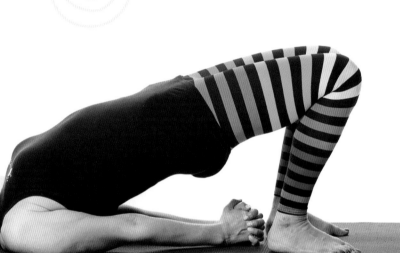

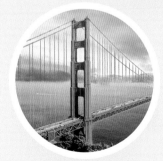

AGE: 3+

POSE TYPE: Backbend

ANATOMICAL FOCUS: Chest, Legs, Back

VALUE: I AM united

Wheel

Urdhva Dhanurasana

WHAT AM I?

In a car, there is **one** of me used for steering, and **four** of me on the bottom.

LET'S MOVE!

Start by lying on your back with your knees bent and your arms extended. Press your hands and feet into the mat and lift your hips up to the sky! **What type of vehicle is your wheel on?**

BEAN TIP: When coming out of Wheel pose remember to tuck your chin into your chest and to lower down **SLOWLY.**

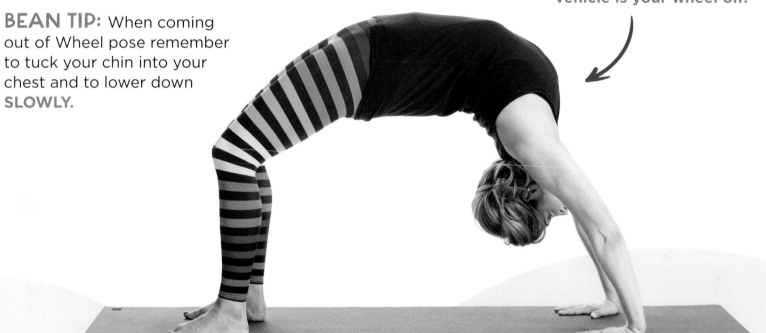

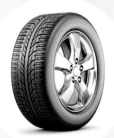

AGE: 5+

POSE TYPE: Backbend

ANATOMICAL FOCUS: Legs, Back

VALUE: I AM energy

HOME SWEET
≈HOME≈

While it is exciting to explore new places, one thing is certain—**there is no place like home.** Being in our favorite room with our special toys is a place that is familiar and makes us feel **safe** and **secure.**

In this chapter, you will get to know the objects that live around you in a whole new way! Get loose like a ragdoll or shine your inner light bright like a candle. **Turn the page,** and let's try it!

Rocking Horse

Dhanurasana

WHAT AM I?

I am a classic **toy** that is shaped like a **horse.** You can sit on me and rock **back-and-forth.**

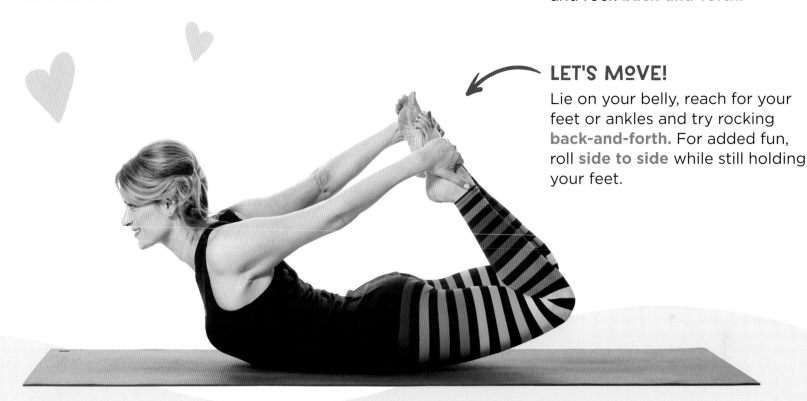

LET'S MOVE!

Lie on your belly, reach for your feet or ankles and try rocking **back-and-forth.** For added fun, roll **side to side** while still holding your feet.

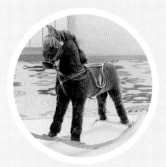

AGE: 5+

POSE TYPE: Backbend

ANATOMICAL FOCUS: Chest, Back

VALUE: I AM imaginative

Candle

Salamba Sarvangasana

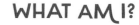

WHAT AM I?

I am made of **wax** with a **wick** in the center. You can put me in a **jack-o-lantern** on Halloween!

BEAN TIP: Remember to always put your body weight on your shoulders and never on your neck.

LET'S MOVE!

From Plow pose (page 30), bend your elbows and place your hands on your back, and then slowly lift your legs up. Use your hands to help **lift** and support your back. **Get creative** and make different shapes with your legs.

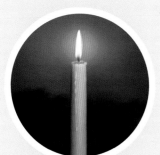

AGE: 5+

POSE TYPE: Inversion

ANATOMICAL FOCUS: Shoulders, Back

VALUE: I AM light

Chair

Utkatasana

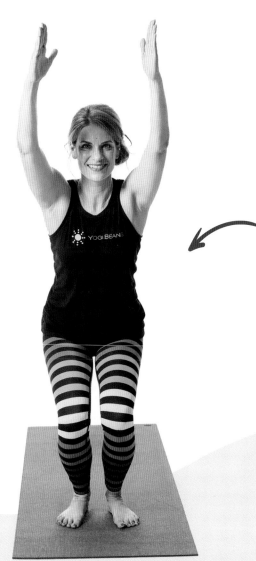

WHAT AM I?

You **sit** on me when you eat at a **table** to have a meal, or when you are at your **desk** at school.

LET'S MOVE!

Bend your knees as you pretend to sit back in an imaginary chair. Lift your arms up above your head. Can you be in a **high chair,** a **low chair** or an **armchair?**

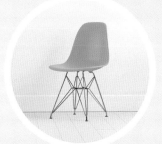

AGE: 3+

POSE TYPE: Standing

ANATOMICAL FOCUS: Legs

VALUE : I AM endurant

Rocking Chair

Utkatasana Variation

WHAT AM I?

I am a type of chair that moves **back and forth.** Babies find me very **calming.**

LET'S MOVE!

From Chair pose (page 115), **bend** your knees and **roll** into a ball on the mat. Try coming back into Chair pose without using your hands to help you stand up!

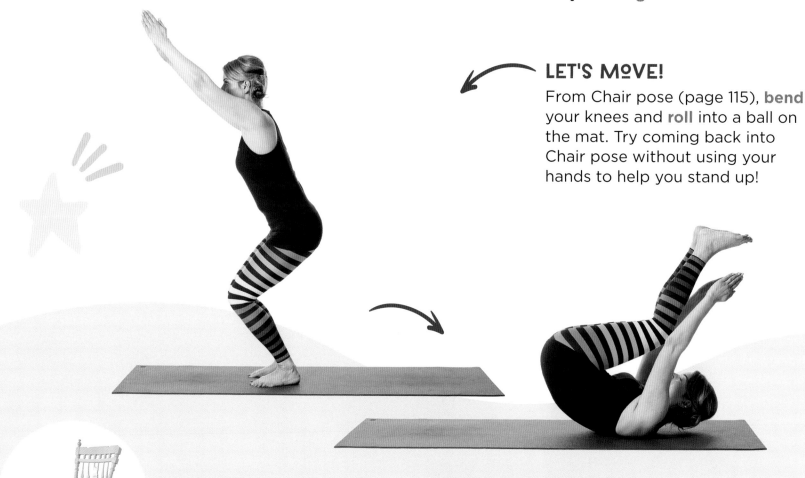

AGE: 5+

POSE TYPE: Standing

ANATOMICAL FOCUS: Legs, Core

VALUE: I AM wholehearted

Swing

Tolasana

BEAN TIP: Place your hands on blocks or books to help lift your seat off the mat more easily.

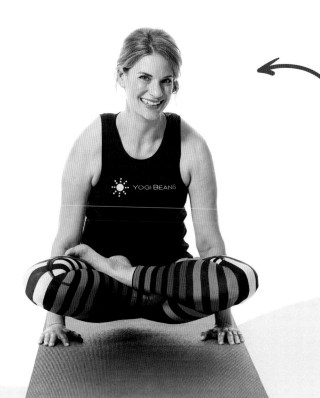

WHAT AM I?

I hang from chains or ropes. If you **sit** on me and **kick** your legs, you will feel as if you are **soaring high** in the sky.

LET'S MOVE!

Begin in Lotus pose (page 56). Bring your hands to the floor outside your thighs. Inhale and **press into your palms;** exhale and lift your legs and bottom off the floor.

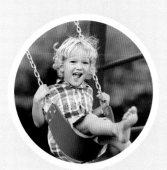

AGE: 5+

POSE TYPE: Arm Balance

ANATOMICAL FOCUS: Core

VALUE: I AM in flow

Slide

Purvottanasana

WHAT AM I?

You can find me at the **playground.** I am fun to go **down** and many children like to climb **up** me too.

LET'S MOVE!

Begin in a Crab pose (page 41) and straighten your legs out in front of you. **For a challenge,** try lifting one leg at a time.

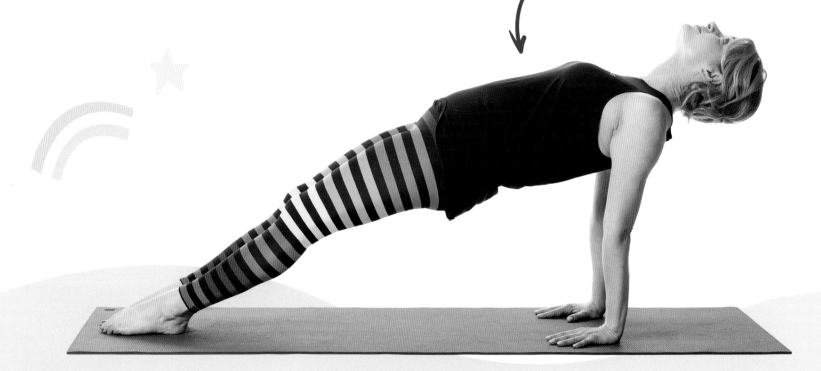

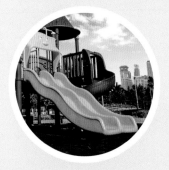

AGE: 5+

POSE TYPE: Core

ANATOMICAL FOCUS: Chest, Core

VALUE: I AM playful

Telephone

Hindolasana Variation

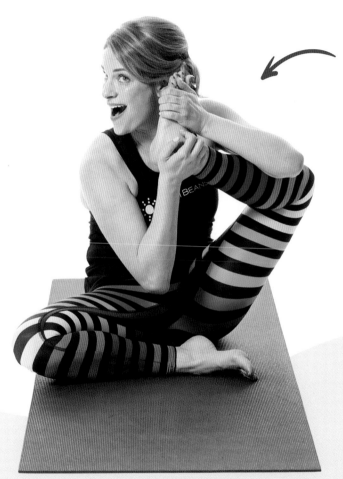

WHAT AM I?

I have the numbers 0 through 9 written on me. **Call me!**

LET'S MOVE!

Sit with your legs crossed, then lift your foot to your ear, or as close as you can get it. **Who is on your phone?** Extend your leg to put your phone on **"speaker"** so everyone can say hello! Don't forget to switch sides.

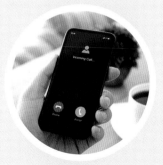

AGE: 2+

POSE TYPE: Hip Opening

ANATOMICAL FOCUS: Legs

VALUE: I AM communicative

Ragdoll

Uttanasana

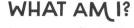

WHAT AM I?

I am a soft **doll** made from **rags** or pieces of **cloth.**

BEAN TIP: Allow your head, shoulders and arms to be loose and relaxed. As you move your head back and forth, shake out any worrisome or negative thoughts.

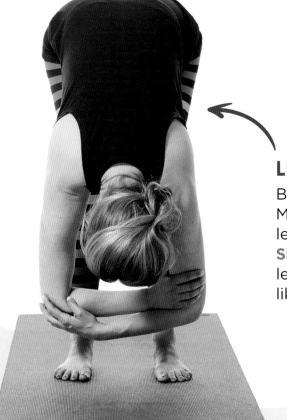

LET'S MOVE!

Begin in Mountain pose (page 19). Melt down over your legs and let your arms **sway** side to side. **Shake** your head side to side and let your body feel **totally loose** like a rag doll.

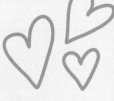

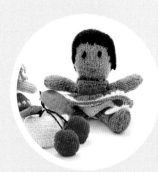

AGE: 2+

POSE TYPE: Forward Bend

ANATOMICAL FOCUS: Legs, Back

VALUE: I AM letting go

Towel

Jathara Parivartanasana

WHAT AM I?

I **dry** you off and keep you **warm** when you get out of the **pool** or **bath.**

LET'S MOVE!

Start lying down on your back with knees bent. Just like we squeeze a towel to get out the water, **twist** your knees to one side and face your head in the opposite direction. Change sides and feel the **deep stretch** to your back.

BEAN TIP: This is a nice pose to do before going into the final resting pose of Savasana (page 137).

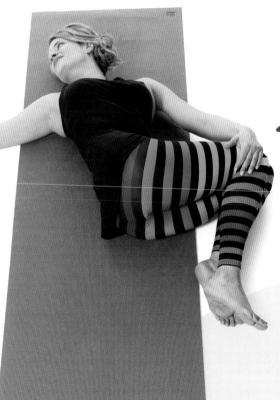

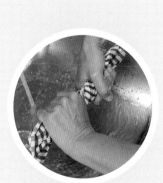

AGE: 3+

POSE TYPE: Twist

ANATOMICAL FOCUS: Back

VALUE: I AM purified

Fan

Prasarita Padottanasana Variation

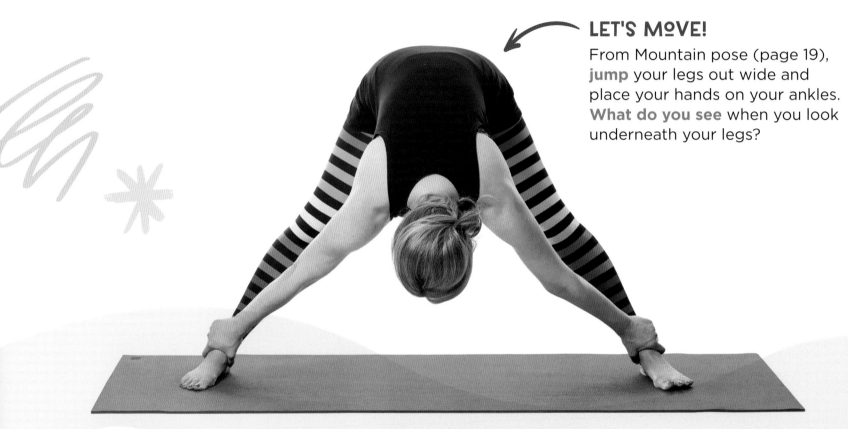

WHAT AM I?

On a **hot** summer day, **wave** me in front of your face to **cool off.**

LET'S MOVE!

From Mountain pose (page 19), **jump** your legs out wide and place your hands on your ankles. **What do you see** when you look underneath your legs?

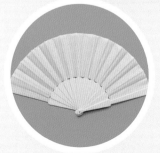

AGE: 2+

POSE TYPE: Forward Bend

ANATOMICAL FOCUS: Legs

VALUE: I AM content

BON
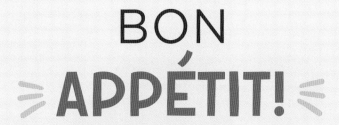
APPÉTIT!

It is time for a snack! Make your favorite **sandwich,** pull some **vegetables** from the garden and enjoy some **sweet treats** as we bend our bodies into **fun food shapes!**

WHAT IS YOUR FAVORITE FOOD?

Banana Split

Parivrtta Janu Sirsasana

WHAT AM I?

I am a classic dessert made up of a **banana**, scoops of **ice cream** and **toppings.**

LET'S MOVE!

Sit with your legs out in front of you in a straddle. Bend one knee and place that foot on the inside of your opposite thigh. **Stretch** your arm into the air to choose your favorite **ice cream** and **toppings.** Fold over your extended leg to add each ingredient to your banana split. Repeat on the other side and you get to enjoy two banana splits!

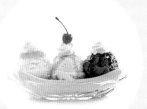

AGE: 3+

POSE TYPE: Seated

ANATOMICAL FOCUS: Legs, Back

VALUE: I AM joyful

Birthday Cake

LET'S MOVE!

In a seated position, follow the images to move your body and make your cake! **(A)** All of your ingredients are on the top shelf. Reach up high to get them! **(B)** Stir the batter. **(C)** Pour the batter in a pan. **(D)** Put it in the oven and let it bake!

WHAT AM I?

Once a year you will put **candles** on me, sing a **song** and then blow out the candles to make a **special wish.**

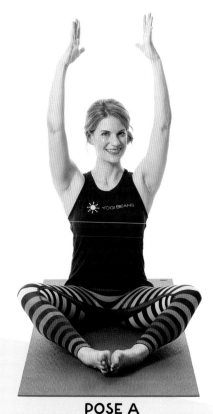

POSE A

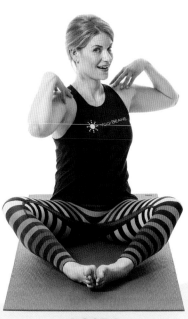

POSE B

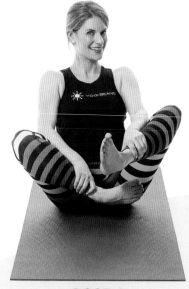

POSE C

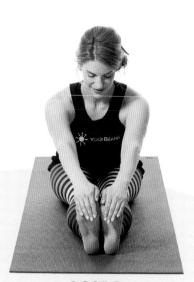

POSE D

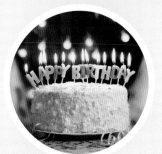

AGE: 3+

POSE TYPE: Seated

ANATOMICAL FOCUS: Legs, Back

VALUE: I AM growing

Yogawich

WHAT AM I?
I am made with two pieces of **bread** and your **favorite foods** in the middle.

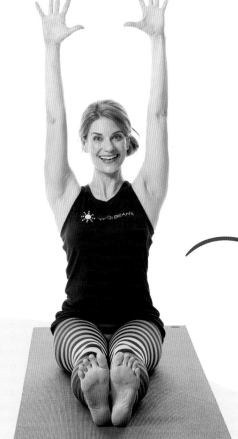

POSE A

POSE B

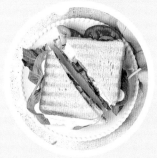

AGE: 2+

POSE TYPE: Forward Bend

ANATOMICAL FOCUS: Legs, Back

VALUE: I AM nourished

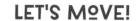

LET'S MOVE!

Imagine your favorite ingredients for your sandwich are in a cabinet. **(A)** Reach up high, to the side and behind to get them. **(B)** Fold over to build your sandwich. **(C)** Cut your sandwich in half by coming into a straddle. **(D)** Bend over and take a bite of both "halves!"

POSE C

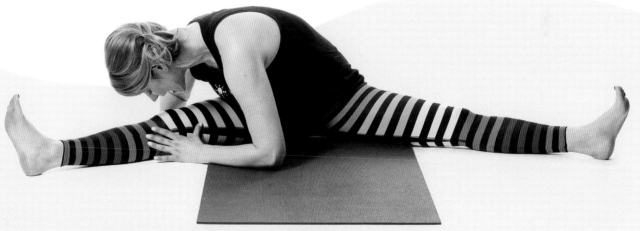

POSE D

Pretzel

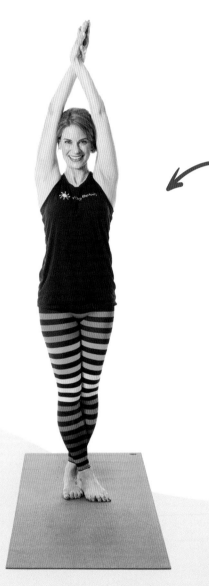

WHAT AM I?

I can be shaped in a **knot, rod or nugget.** Some people think I taste best with mustard.

LET'S MOVE!

Stand tall with your hands above your head and cross your hands and your ankles. **Take a "bite"** of the pretzel by taking a side stretch to one side and then to the other.

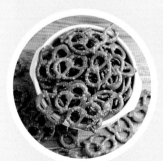

AGE: 2+

POSE TYPE: Standing

ANATOMICAL FOCUS: Legs, Arms

VALUE: I AM grateful

Carrot

Supta Padangusthasana Variation

WHAT AM I?

I am a root vegetable that is usually **orange.** I am loved by **rabbits, horses** and **people!**

LET'S MOVE!

Lie on your back and extend one leg up vertically. Reach for your extended leg and gently pull your leg toward you as if you were pulling a **carrot** out of the **soil.** Switch to the other leg to pull another carrot!

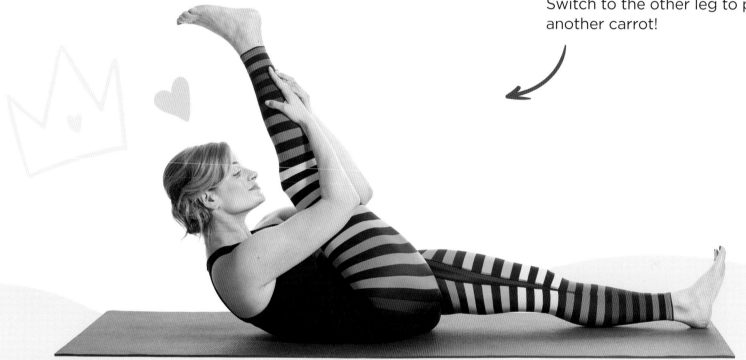

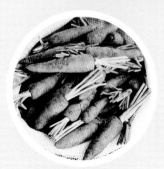

AGE: 3+

POSE TYPE: Supine

ANATOMICAL FOCUS: Legs

VALUE: I AM rooted

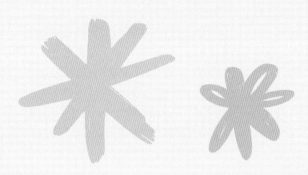

PARTNER POSES

LET'S DOUBLE THE FUN!

Find a buddy you trust and **practice** these poses **together!**
Remember to **communicate** with each other how each pose feels
(too much, too little). Most importantly, **have fun!**

Double Down

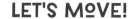

LET'S MOVE!

Stand back-to-back with your partner and come into Downward Dog pose (page 13). One partner remains in Downward Dog while the other partner lifts one leg at a time so that the tops of their feet are resting on their partner's lower back, right above their tailbone. The partner on the ground keeps their arms strong. **No floppy spaghetti arms!**

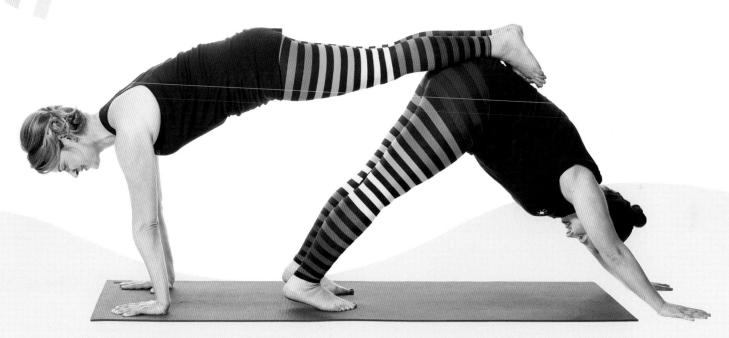

AGE: 5+

POSE TYPE: Partner Inversion

ANATOMICAL FOCUS: Legs, Core

VALUE: WE ARE strong

Partner Boat / Flower

LET'S MOVE!

With your partner, press your feet into one another while holding hands. Next, bring both your feet in between your arms for Partner Boat **(A)**. Then, bend your knees and bring your legs outside your arms for a Partner Flower **(B)**. **Have fun moving between the two poses!**

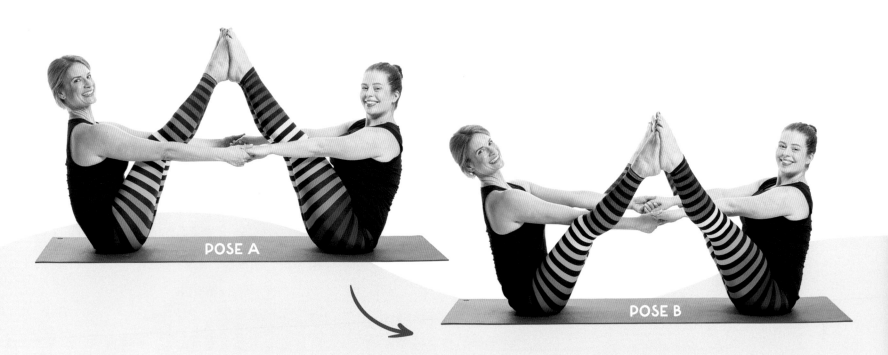

POSE A

POSE B

AGE: 5+

POSE TYPE: Partner Seated (Front to Front)

ANATOMICAL FOCUS: Legs, Core

VALUE: WE ARE coordinated

Partner Armchairs

LET'S MOVE!

Start sitting with your knees bent. Press your backs into each other and lock arms to become one chair. **Support each other** as you rise in **harmony.**

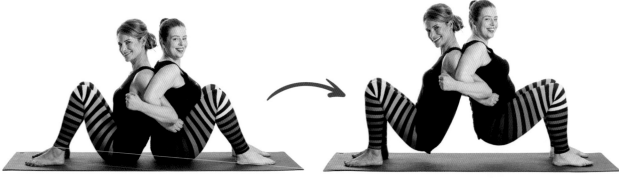

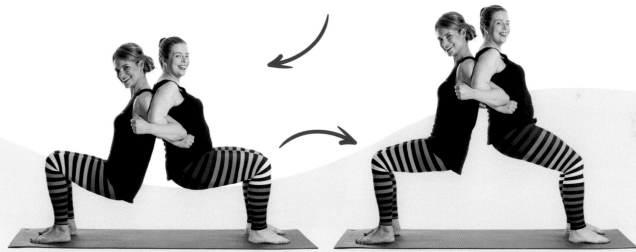

AGE: 5+

POSE TYPE: Partner Seated (Back to Back)

ANATOMICAL FOCUS: Legs, Core

VALUE: WE ARE united

Whirlpool

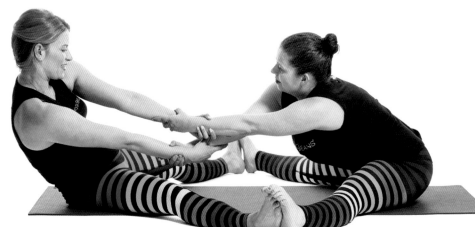

LET'S MOVE!

Face your partner in a seated straddle and **press** your feet together. **Cross** your arms and **hold** hands. Now, to make the whirlpool, **circle** your upper bodies in opposite directions so one partner is learning forward while the other partner is leaning backward. Practice picking up speed and then switching directions.

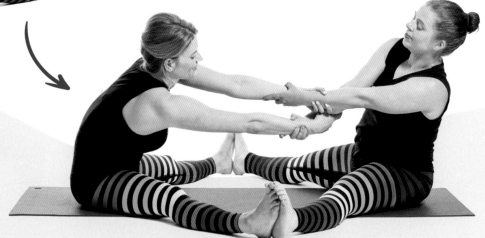

AGE: 5+

POSE TYPE: Partner Seated (Front to Front)

ANATOMICAL FOCUS: Back

VALUE: WE ARE energy

Golden Gates

LET'S MOVE!

Stand on one knee with the other extended long to the side, crossed with your partner's leg.

Bend to the side and bring your hands to meet in the middle of your gate. In sync with your breath, practice opening and closing the gate.

For more fun, add a secret **password** or **phrase** to open the gate.

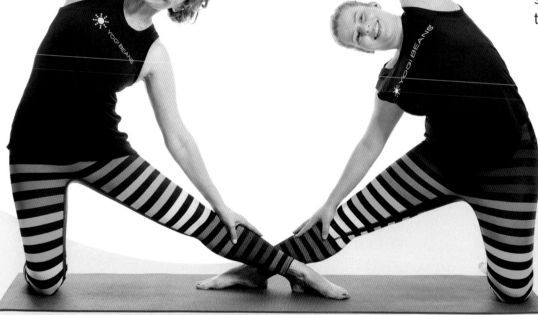

AGE: 3+

ANATOMICAL FOCUS: Core

POSE TYPE: Partner Standing (Side to Side)

VALUE: WE ARE connected

FINAL RESTING POSE
SAVASANA

Last, and certainly not least, is the final resting pose called Savasana. Some people refer to Savasana as the most important pose. It is a time for your body to **rest, relax** and **absorb** the benefits of your practice.

Savasana

BEAN TIP: It can be nice to listen to your favorite relaxing song while resting in Savasana.

LET'S NOT MOVE!

Lie down on your back. You may choose to close your eyes. It can be helpful to place your hand on your heart or belly to **connect** to your breath. Allow your body to **melt** into the mat as if you were ice cream melting on a hot summer day. Rest in this pose for 1 to 3 minutes or longer.

You can **repeat the following meditation** in your mind as you lie in Savasana:

**MAY I BE HAPPY. MAY I BE HEALTHY.
MAY I BE KIND. MAY I BE CARING.
MAY I BE SAFE. MAY I BE LOVED.
MAY I KNOW THAT ALL IS WELL.**

When it is time to come out of Savasana, gently wiggle your fingers and toes, bring your knees to your chest and give yourself a hug. Take a deep breath and thank yourself for making time to take care of your **body, mind** and **heart.**

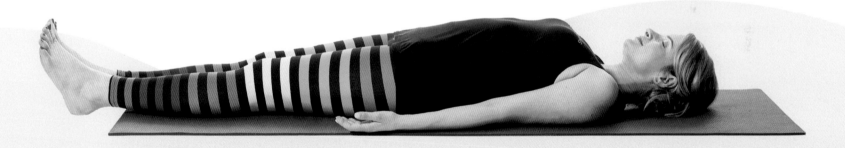

AGE: All

POSE TYPE: Restorative

ANATOMICAL FOCUS: Full Body

VALUE: I AM relaxed

Glossary

Asana (ah-suh-nuh): The Sanskrit word for seat or pose.

Ayurveda (ah-yer-vey-duh): Translated literally from Sanskrit as "science of life," Ayurveda is a natural system of medicine that originated in India more than 3,000 years ago.

Drishti (dr-ishti): A focused gaze to help enhance concentration. The use of drishti is often used during asana, pranayama and meditation to help obtain one pointed focus and attention.

Mala (ma-la): A string of beads that can be used during meditation to count prayers or mantras. *Mala* is Sanskrit for rosary or garland.

Mantra (muhn-truh): A word or sound repeated to help with meditation and concentration.

Namaste (nuhm-uh-stey): A traditional Hindu greeting of deep respect, which directly translates to "I bow to you." The gesture associated with Namaste is to bring the hands together in front of the heart and bow the head. Namaste is often used at the end of a yoga class.

Pranayama (pran-a-ya-ma): The yogic practice of focusing on the breath. In Sanskrit, *prana* is defined as "life force energy" and *yama* means "to control." So, pranayama can be defined as controlling life force energy.

Sanskrit (san-skrit): The religious and classical language of India that has been in use since 1200 BC.

Vedic (vey-dik): In relation to the Vedas, the entire body of Hindu sacred writings.

Yoga (yoh-guh): The word "yoga" can be translated to mean "union" and is defined as the union of the mind and the self.

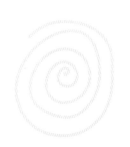

Acknowledgments

Our first debt of gratitude is to Sarah Monroe, our editor at Page Street Publishing. Thank you for enduring the reading of our manuscript full of roaring lions and barking seals more than once! And for your expert notes and invaluable guidance.

To William Kiester, publisher of Page Street Publishing: Thank you for offering us a new home. Thank you to the entire Page Street book publishing team for your creative suggestions, honesty and advice.

Thank you to our agent Liz Nealon of Great Dog Literary who helped us navigate the literary world with extraordinary perspicacity and determination. You saw our vision and helped us craft our story—we are authors only because of you!

Where words can do no justice, we owe Jonathan Hollingsworth much appreciation for referring us to our agent and for being a marvelous friend.

Lashaun Dale, our genie: You are a visionary and mastermind of program and brand strategy. We are forever appreciative of your help unlocking the magic of Yogi Beans.

Thank you to our parents who supported our creative endeavors since we were both little Beans. We pass on that same unconditional support to our daughters, Vivienne and Juliette, who inspire us daily with their creativity and imagination.

In countless ways, many people who positively change the lives of children contributed to this book. To our instructors, the Bean Team, and all the parents, educators and partners that we work with: We send you our heartfelt thanks for your support and belief in children's unbound human potential!

About Yogi Beans

Yogi Beans is the brainchild of Lauren and Brian Chaitoff. In 2007, they founded a novel yoga curriculum for children and began offering classes to the public at various schools, yoga studios and other venues throughout New York City. After becoming parents in 2013, Lauren and Brian became more strongly dedicated to supporting children and their well-being. Their mission has always been to help children everywhere grow healthier and happier—for life!

Lauren is the face of Yogi Beans and embodies the new age of mind-body fitness. She was first introduced to yoga and Pilates as a theater major at Northwestern University. Upon graduation, she received her Pilates certification through the PhysicalMind Institute and Master Trainer Ivon Dahl. After moving back to New York City, Lauren completed her 200-hour yoga certification through YogaWorks and became a registered E–RYT Yoga Instructor and member of the Yoga Alliance.

Lauren is a champion of spreading awareness of yoga's effectiveness at stress reduction and emotional regulation in children. Her exemplary work has been featured on *Good Morning America*, ABC News, the *New York Post* and in other publications.

Brian handles the operating business of Yogi Beans and focuses on growth and product expansion. After graduating with a degree in business administration (BSBA) from Boston University, Brian spent time at a preeminent law firm in New York City before sailing off into the venture world where he worked at alternative data startups over the following years.

Today, Yogi Beans is a 16-year leader in the children's yoga and wellness industry. We deliver wellness education through yoga, mindfulness programming and transformative wellness experiences for babies to teens and those who love them. Our programs are streamed worldwide through omstars.com and experienced through our partners including American Girl, Rosewood Hotels & Resorts, Athleta, the NYC Department of Education and many other leaders.

At Yogi Beans, everything we do—our books, classes, digital programs, trainings, events and advocacy—are focused on children and those who support and raise them every day. To do this, we educate and cultivate the whole child, their families and their communities.

Lauren and Brian reside in Long Island, New York, with their two daughters, Vivienne and Juliette, and their dog Buddha.

Visit us at yogibeans.com.

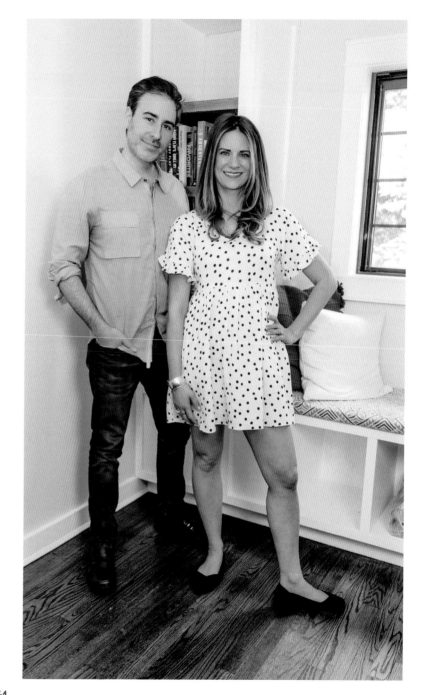

Index